Smart Sourdough

The No-Starter, No-Waste, No-Cheat, No-Fail Way to Make Naturally Fermented Bread in 24 Hours or Less with Your Home Proofer, Instant Pot, Slow Cooker, Sous Vide Cooker, or Other Warmer

— Mark Shepard —

There's sourdough, and then there's *smart* sourdough—a whole new approach to an ancient bread!

Most sourdough recipes lead you through days or even weeks of developing a starter before you can make your bread—and then into a lifetime of maintaining that starter. But this book is based on the belief that all that rigmarole is no longer needed. With modern methods of regulating temperature, and with the easy availability of baker's yeast, honest-to-goodness naturally fermented sourdough bread can be made from start to finish in less than a day.

With all the benefits of naturally fermented sourdough, it's only the hassle of making it that has discouraged home bakers. Well, hassle no more. The age of smart sourdough has arrived.

Books by Mark Shepard

Cookbooks

Smart Sourdough

Simple Sourdough

Music

How to Love Your Flute

Simple Flutes

Alternatives

Gandhi Today

The Community of the Ark

Mahatma Gandhi and His Myths

Poetry

Songs of Flesh, Songs of Spirit

Smart Sourdough

The No-Starter, No-Waste, No-Cheat, No-Fail Way to Make Naturally Fermented Bread in 24 Hours or Less with Your Home Proofer, Instant Pot, Slow Cooker, Sous Vide Cooker, or Other Warmer

Mark Shepard

Foreword by Anne L. Watson

Shepard Publications
Bellingham, Washington

Library of Congress Control Number: 2020939996
Library of Congress subject headings: Cookery (Sourdough), Baking, Bread

Version 1.0

Acknowledgments

Though the method described in this book is strictly my own, it has benefited a great deal from the publicly shared knowledge of many bakers, fermenters, and scientists. Special thanks go to Michael G. Gänzle, Daniel Wing, Debra Wink, Kurt Janz, Sandor Ellix Katz, Peter Reinhart, Ken Forkish, Stanley Ginsberg, William Alexander, the cooks at America's Test Kitchen, and Rob Dunn, Anne Madden, and the other researchers of the Sourdough Project.

Thanks for valuable feedback go to Pamela O. Lilley, Kirsten and Christopher Shockey, and the commenters in The Fresh Loaf forum.

Above all, thanks to my beloved wife, Anne L. Watson, who along with testing provided support, suggestions, and most crucially, tasting.

Cover Photos

Front cover, top: Sliced loaf of smart sourdough
Front cover, bottom: Warming devices for smart sourdough
Back cover, first row left: Double large round loaf of smart sourdough
Back cover, first row right: A lunch with fermented foods
Back cover, second row left: Mark's Sourdough Skillet Pizza
Back cover, second row center top: Smart Mediterranean Sourdough
Back cover, second row center bottom: Tin figure painted by Anne L. Watson
Back cover, second row right: Mark's Masala Dosa
Back cover, third row left: Essential ingredients of smart sourdough
Back cover, third row right: NutriMill Classic
Back cover, fourth row: Sourdough bread bowl with clam chowder

Please do not eat raw dough—sourdough or otherwise!

Contents

Foreword
by Anne L. Watson

I first encountered sourdough bread when I was a college student in San Francisco. I thought of it as restaurant fare, not something I'd consider making at home.

Not then. Many years later, I decided to give it a try. I ordered San Francisco Sourdough Starter online and followed the directions. I don't remember the exact procedure, but it was rather like having a pet of some kind stashed in the refrigerator, requiring daily attention and care. Finally, I got to make my bread.

It was a complete failure.

Now, I have to admit to a bit of vanity about my breadmaking skills. I've been making various kinds of yeast bread ever since my sister and I, at ages 14 and 12, discovered a pizza recipe in a kids' cookbook. So, I was more than a little annoyed when that

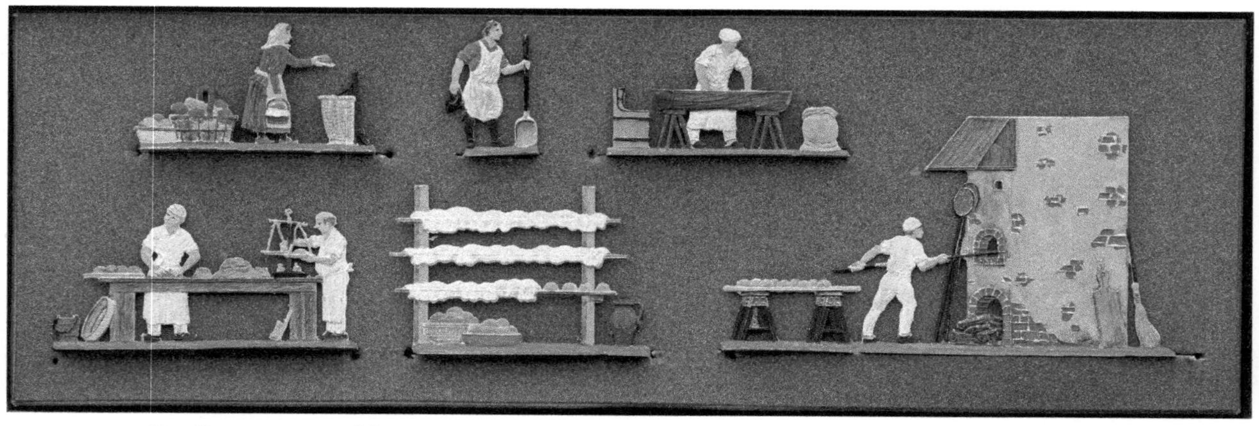

Tin figures painted by Anne L. Watson. From the set Medieval Bakery by the German manufacturer Maier, depicting a European bakery of the 1700s. Pewter alloy, at a scale of 30 millimeters (1.2 inches, the height of the human figures), shown here at half size.

sourdough didn't work for me. I threw out my costly starter and dismissed sourdough as one of those things like puff pastry or dim sum that I was just going to have to buy if I wanted it.

Then Mark started working on his new approach to sourdough. I liked his idea of not coping with a starter stored in the refrigerator, but when I tried the results of his earliest methods, I liked my yeast bread better. Months went by, and from time to time, he'd have me taste samples from his experiments. At first, they weren't impressive. And then . . .

And then he perfected a technique he describes in this book, his method of no-waste feedings. Suddenly, the bread was delicious—different from the bread I remembered from my student days, but at least that good. I knew, though, what an expert he'd become in getting to that point, and I doubted it would work for me.

But I tried it. The bread was perfect. And I didn't even have to go to San Francisco for it.

Anne L. Watson is the author of the Smart Soapmaking series, the Smart Housekeeping series, and two books on baking with cookie molds, as well as many literary novels and children's picture books. She lives in Bellingham, Washington, with her sourdough-making husband. Visit her at www.annelwatson.com.

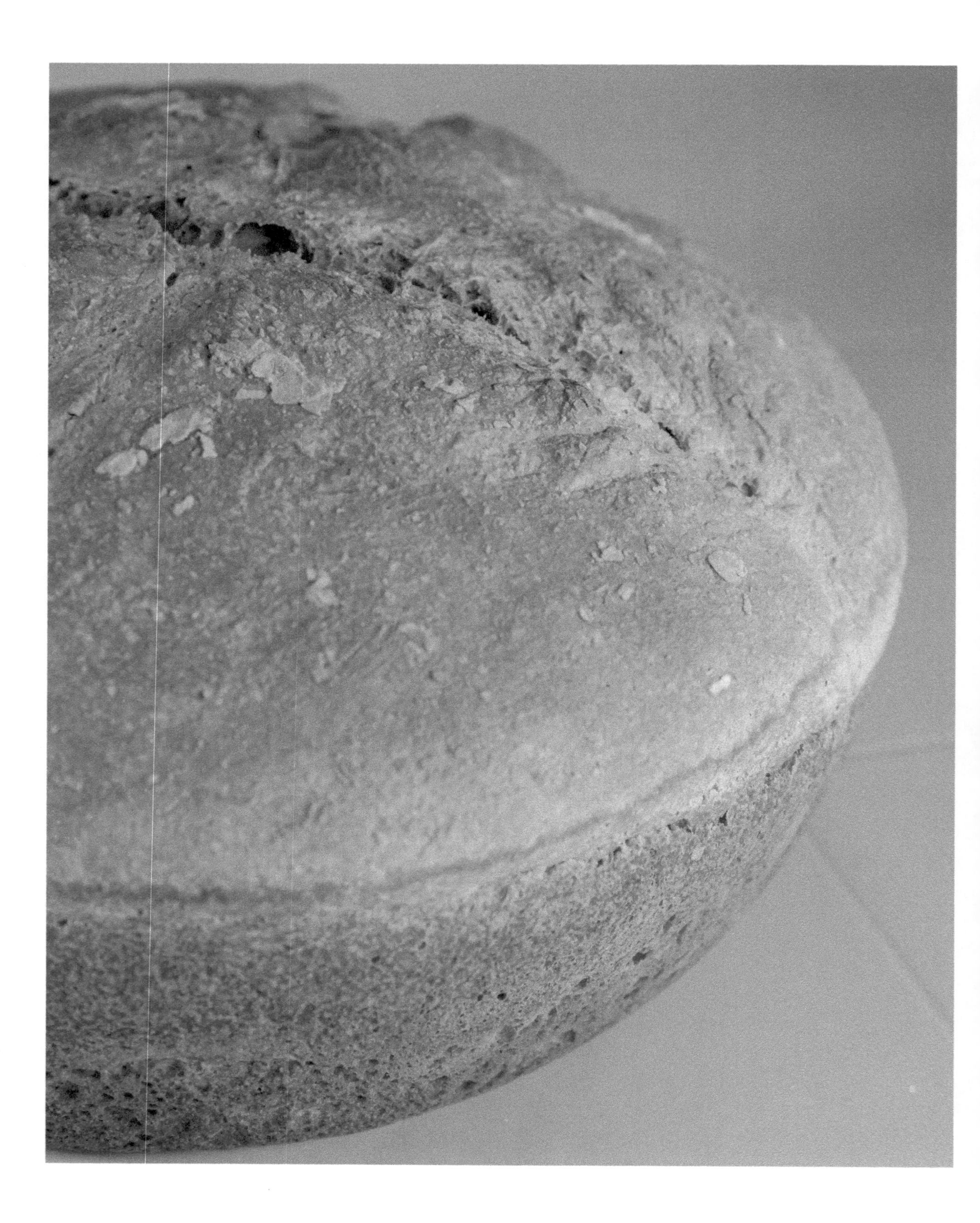

Getting Started

If you've never made sourdough before, you'll be surprised how simple it can be. And if you *have* made sourdough before, you may be even *more* surprised!

Most sourdough recipes lead you through days or even weeks of developing a starter before you can make your bread—and then into a lifetime of maintaining that starter. But this book is based on the belief that all that rigmarole is no longer needed. With modern methods of regulating temperature, and with the easy availability of (*gasp!*) baker's yeast, honest-to-goodness naturally fermented sourdough bread can be made from start to finish in less than a day.

Let me explain. Though sourdough bakers often talk about collecting "wild yeast" in their starters, what they're actually trying to collect is a combination of yeast and bacteria—a special kind called *lactic acid bacteria*, named after the main acid they give off.

If the name *lactic acid* sounds exotic or intimidating, it doesn't have to. It's what creates sourness or tang in sour cream, yogurt, and many other milk products—which is why it's called *lactic*, or "related to milk." It's also the main source of sourness in pickles and sauerkraut whenever they're naturally fermented instead of made with vinegar.

All those foods are produced with bacteria of the same family found in sourdough. And it's these bacteria, rather than any kind of yeast, that make sourdough what it is.

In case you have any doubt about that, consider these advantages of making naturally fermented sourdough over making conventional yeast bread:

• Gives the bread a delicious sourness or tang.

• Weakens the gluten, making it easier to digest for people who might otherwise have trouble with it.

• Adds acids that slow the digestion of starches, for a lower glycemic index and improved blood sugar response.

• Reduces amounts of antinutrients like phytic acid and lectins, making nutrients in the flour more available to you.

• Resists spoilage in the baked bread and keeps it fresher longer.

Every one of these advantages is produced chiefly or entirely by the sourdough bacteria, not the sourdough yeast. And the one job that *is* chiefly handled by the sourdough yeast—making the bread rise—is done *as well or better* by baker's yeast.

That being true, why worry about sourdough yeast at all? A good part of the labor of traditional sourdough is keeping the yeast going strong in a starter. In place of that, why not focus on nurturing the bacteria and just add a bit of baker's yeast at the end? Not so strangely, that's exactly how sourdough is made today in many commercial bakeries!

And there's more. With yeast out of the equation, it turns out you can get flour to ferment very quickly, even from scratch. So quickly, in fact, *you don't need a starter at all.* Just add water to high-quality whole grain flour, keep the mixture at a good temperature for a matter of hours, and occasionally add more flour. You'll get sourdough every time.

With all the benefits of naturally fermented sourdough, it's only the hassle of making it that has discouraged home bakers. Well, hassle no more. The age of smart sourdough has arrived.

Sourdough Superstitions

Before tackling how to make smart sourdough, let's demolish some half-truths and outright falsehoods that might stand in our way. (I'll discuss many of these later in the book in more detail.)

Myth: Sourdough is very sour!

Some sourdough *is* very sour—for instance, the kind popularly associated with San Francisco. But the *sour* in *sourdough* really only means the dough is fermented by lactic acid bacteria. These bacteria produce both acetic acid, which tastes more sour, and lactic acid, which tastes less so—and how you make the bread helps decide the amounts and proportions of these two acids. That's why, for instance, you'll hear of the "sweet" sourdoughs of Italy in contrast to the more sour ones of Germany.

With the 24-hour process described here, the sourness will be milder and the taste more complex than in a typical San Francisco sourdough. In fact, you might find your bread turns out more tangy than sour. That's okay, and you may well prefer it! But I'll also give you simple tips for turning the sourness up or down—and in any case, you'll get all the benefits of sourdough, including improved taste, however "sweet" or sour that may be.

Myth: Sourdough takes a lot of work!

What takes a lot of work is beginning and maintaining a traditional sourdough starter. But with modern methods of temperature control, plus the judicious use of a tiny amount of baker's yeast at the end, making naturally fermented sourdough doesn't require a starter at all. It's still a bit more work than making regular yeast bread, but the health benefits—and taste!—are well worth it.

Myth: When you start sourdough, there's always the risk it will go bad and have to be thrown out.

That's with traditional sourdough starter, and it's because the starter is fermenting at around room temperature. The higher temperatures of smart sourdough favor the bacteria you want, so it's easy for them to overcome their undesirable competitors.

I call this method no-fail because a mixture of high-quality whole grain flour and water at the temperatures I recommend will *always* go properly sour. There *is* some risk of it going bad later from being pushed too far, but I'll teach you how to control that. In fact, since perfecting my recipe, *I have not had a single batch of sourdough go bad on me*, though each and every one has been started from scratch.

Myth: Sourdough is wasteful because you have to discard so much when you feed it.

Making and maintaining a traditional starter can certainly be wasteful, since you're typically told to discard as much as half the sourdough before feeding. Of course, you can find other uses for the sourdough you've removed, but that can be a hassle in itself.

With smart sourdough, *none* is discarded. You simply start with a very wet sponge, then let each feeding bring it closer to the moisture content of a finished loaf. No more conflict between conscience and convenience!

Myth: Sourdough was the first risen bread.

This is technically true but also misleading. Sourdough bakers often make this claim to conjure images of ancient bakers nurturing their precious and delicate starters. But that is almost certainly *not* how bread was first fermented. In a hot and humid climate like in Egypt—where risen bread is said to have first appeared—all you need to ferment dough is to leave it overnight.

Of course, it would have been natural for some Egyptian bakers to start saving a bit of dough from one batch to speed up fermenting in another. But it wasn't until sourdough moved to the cooler climes of Europe that bakers needed elaborate procedures for developing and maintaining starters. European bakers had no way to maintain the kind of temperatures common where sourdough originated, so they had to come up with alternative methods. This is the approach that bread historians and technologists now call Type I sourdough. (That's a Roman numeral 1.)

Type I is what many bakers today think of as the only *true* sourdough, even though it was dictated only by practical necessity in certain parts of the world at a certain time in history—a time that is now past.

Myth: With sourdough, the starter provides the leavening.

That's true of Type I sourdough. But much of the sourdough sold today—especially by supermarkets and large bakeries—is what we call Type II (Roman numeral 2). The dough is fermented by sourdough bacteria, but yeast growth is actually discouraged till the end, when baker's yeast is added for the rise.

Development of this technology began in the late 20th century. But most home bakers—and cooking writers—have yet to hear of this new approach, much less to absorb its lessons. Though Type II itself is an industrial process suited only to large bakeries, this book aims to adapt some of its principles to the home kitchen.

Myth: You need a starter so you don't have to start your sourdough from scratch each time.

A starter will certainly do this for you, but it no longer matters so much. With modern temperature control, you can easily ferment your flour from scratch in less than a day. You won't get the traditional balance of yeast and bacteria in that time, but you don't need to, because you can just add a bit of baker's yeast at the end. So, you can easily do without a starter.

Of course, there's nothing *wrong* with using a starter. A starter can be helpful if you're making loaves every day or so and want to shorten the time for each one, or if you need to ensure a specific taste—especially a more sour one—or if you just want greater control of your results.

But just to ferment your dough for health and great taste? No, you don't need one. And for most home bakers, they're more trouble than they're worth.

Myth: Bread isn't truly sourdough unless it's made only with wild yeast.

This is kind of a joke, because when scientists studied artisan bakeries in different countries, most of them turned out to have baker's yeast in their sourdough starters! They can't help it. Since these bakeries use baker's yeast for *other* breads and baked goods, it's all over their kitchens and inevitably winds up in their starters.

The results were even more stark in a study of 500 starters from amateur and pro bakers around the world. Baker's yeast dominated an astounding 92% of those starters—including ones in countries where that yeast species had never been found in the wild. Of course, most owners of those starters *thought* they were leavening with wild yeast!

Then there are cooking writers. You know those photos in books, articles, and blog posts that show how easily you can harness wild yeast to make a bubbly starter in just a day or two? What they *really* show is how the writers collected baker's yeast that was hanging around their kitchens. Well, sure, *that's* easy enough! Nurturing *wild* yeast to the point it can raise bread takes at least a few days longer.

In any case, it's bacteria, not yeast, that put the *sour* in *sourdough*. What kind of yeast you're using, and where it came from, doesn't make any difference in that.

Myth: The best way to start sourdough is to add grapes or potato peels or . . .

Ever heard the phrase "carrying coals to Newcastle"? There's no need to add anything extra to your sourdough, or to expose it to the air, either. All the sourdough microbes you need are on the wheat as it was grown. And doesn't it make sense that microbes suited to fermenting your flour would be among those already on the grain?

What you *do* need, though, is some amount of *whole* wheat or another whole grain in your flour. Those sourdough microbes live on the outer surface of the grain, and if that surface is removed—as in most commercial milling—most or all of the microbes go with it. The flour from what's left will probably still ferment, but it can take much longer, and it might not develop as you want.

A variation of this myth is that you should add some rye flour. Sure, rye is great at supplying sourdough microbes—but mainly because it's a whole grain, not because it's rye! Whole wheat flour—as long as it's not overly processed—should work about as well.

Myth: Frothy bubbles mean the sourdough is gaining strength.

Unless you're working with a mature starter, with lots of yeast growing in it, bubbles more likely mean your bacteria have begun a death spiral. When sourdough bacteria are on the rise, they use the food on hand to grow and multiply, producing lactic acid as a by-product, with little visible sign of their activity. When their food runs low, they start sputtering and spewing out acetic acid and carbon dioxide—the gas that makes the bubbles.

That means they're just one step away from running out of food and going dormant or flat-out dying. And if they die and start to decompose? Well, then you get the putrid smell that many sourdough bakers encounter a day or two into making a starter—just when they think it has begun to take off!

Myth: Salt retards sourdough, so you should add it only at the end.

Salt does slightly retard the growth of sourdough microbes—but it retards the growth of *other* microbes even more. The cumulative effect is to *help* the sourdough microbes, reducing competition and allowing them to dominate more quickly. Salt, then, should be added as early as possible!

Myth: Sourdough bacteria are more active at lower temperatures.

The best temperatures for sourdough bacteria are actually above 86°F (30°C)—higher than for most sourdough yeast. But there's a good reason this myth is so widely believed. When sourdough bacteria are forced to live at lower temperatures, they get stressed, and when they get stressed, they produce less lactic acid and more acetic acid. Since acetic acid tastes and smells stronger than lactic does, it's easy to (falsely) conclude that the bacteria are more active at these temperatures.

Myth: It's dangerous to warm any food for long because harmful bacteria can grow.

For meat and cooked foods, this is certainly true. But moderately heating a mixture of flour and water encourages healthful microbes to dominate unhealthful ones. This is much the same way milk is preserved by fermenting it into yogurt, or cabbage by fermenting it into sauerkraut.

Fermenting of plant-based foods is actually considered one of the safest ways to preserve them. The danger from bad microbes is much higher in canning. That's because the heat in canning kills off *all* beneficial microbes, leaving no competition for the bad ones, which are more likely to survive extremely high temperatures and which thrive in the airless environment of the sealed container. So, it's not uncommon to hear of people dying from canned food, while you won't hear the same about sourdough!

Myth: Sourdough may be delicious, but gluten is bad for you.

No, gluten is a wonderful source of protein that has served humanity well for thousands of years. It's true that people with celiac disease really should have no gluten at all—but that's only about 1% of everyone. For others, if there's any real problem, it's likely to be with modern-day chemical additives that toughen gluten so that factories can make bread that's mostly air.

You might get some of those same chemicals in instant or rapid-rise yeast. So, if you're concerned, just avoid those kinds in your baking.

Myth: Maybe gluten is okay, but what about lectins?

Not all lectins are bad—some are important for health—and few of us get enough bad ones in our diets to account for all the problems now claimed for them. Anyway, if you want to worry about lectins, making sourdough is a perfect way to deal with them, because fermenting destroys most of them.

Who's Afraid of Baker's Yeast?

Probably this book's most controversial advice is to add baker's yeast to your sourdough for the rise. Actually, this practice is common in artisan bakeries, where there's even a name for it: "spiking the dough." But to many home sourdough bakers, the idea is heresy, pure and simple. So, it's worth saying a few more words about it.

Truthfully, before I started research and testing for this book, I would *never* have considered adding commercial yeast to my sourdough. To me, that was the worst kind of sourdough cheating. But the more I learned, the more I had to question my bias.

My belief that baker's yeast is a recent invention turned out to be mostly wrong. The yeast species used in commercial baker's yeast—*Saccharomyces cerevisiae*, if you want to get technical—is the same species used for thousands of years to brew beer. Food historians say at least some ancient Egyptian bakers probably leavened their bread with yeast of this kind, which they obtained from breweries. We know for a fact this is how bakeries in the United States got yeast for their bread in the 1800s.

What we call *brewer's yeast* today, though, was later bred from certain *strains* of that species—strains that were suited more to brewing and less to baking. In response to that, food scientists developed *baker's yeast* from strains of the same species but with the opposite character. So, yes, the product known as baker's yeast is relatively new, but it's a refinement of something used by bakers for millennia.

I also had to give up my belief that baker's yeast was somehow inferior to natural yeast. First of all, baker's yeast *is* a natural yeast, as are *all* yeasts. *Saccharomyces cerevisiae* is also found in nature. The only difference in commercial strains is that they have been isolated and bred for greater strength. This is not very different from what sourdough bakers do when they develop a starter to encourage some strains of yeast and bacteria and discourage others. And no one claims that these yeasts or bacteria are less "natural" if you add them as dried bits from someone else's starter you bought online.

With that understood, I couldn't deny that baker's yeast is mostly *superior* to other yeast species found in sourdough. It's stronger, making the bread rise faster and higher. That's why this one species has been isolated and cultivated!

What makes sourdough superior to other bread is the sourdough *bacteria*. It's these bacteria that mostly produce each advantage of sourdough—while the relative weakness of most sourdough yeast species may be this bread's most common *dis*advantage.

The fact is, if using cultivated yeast bothers you, then you probably shouldn't be eating wheat either. All modern wheat is a product of continual breeding from older species of wild grass—there's not a single wheat variety that comes directly from nature. So, baker's yeast is *at least* as natural as wheat itself.

In the end, all these facts and thoughts raised for me an unavoidable question: Why not? If it would entirely get rid of my need for a starter while still making my dough double in volume, why shouldn't I add a pinch or two of yeast?

I couldn't think of a single good reason. Can you?

The Right Ingredients

Smart sourdough is more an approach than a specific recipe. So, to start you off, we'll keep the ingredients basic: just flour, water, salt, and yeast.

Those are really all you need to make a delicious, nutritious, satisfying loaf. In fact, that's all I put in the basic bread I eat every day. Sourdough with more ingredients is something I make more as a treat.

But despite smart sourdough having so few essential ingredients—or maybe because of it—there's a fair amount to say about each.

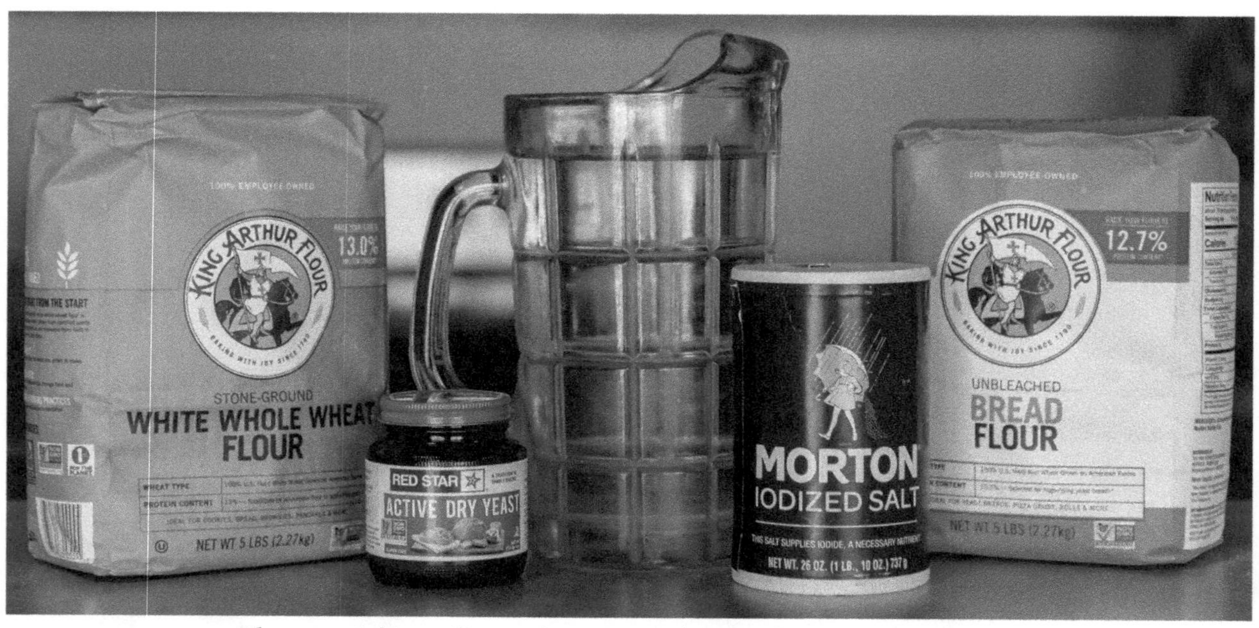

The essential ingredients of smart sourdough—flour, water, salt, yeast

Flour

You probably know that most wheat flour today is produced by removing the bran and the germ from the wheat kernel, giving us what's commonly called white flour. You probably also know that this provides longer shelf life and better rise, but at the expense of most of the wheat's flavor and nutrition.

That alone is enough reason to use whole wheat flour in place of at least some of the white flour in our bread. But with sourdough, there's another reason: *The parts removed from white flour contain most of the microbes that can ferment the grain.* While it's possible to get those microbes elsewhere, the quickest and most efficient source is the flour itself. And that's important when trying to make sourdough from scratch within 24 hours!

Other whole grains, like rye, are also good for supplying microbes—but for our basic recipe, we'll stick to wheat. All whole wheat flour, though, is not created equal! The brand you choose can make a huge difference in your sourdough.

Probably the *worst* brand you can choose is a cheap one from the baking section of your supermarket. Any whole wheat flour produced for economy is bound to be made from less desirable wheat and processed with less regard for preserving nutrition. It's likely to contain more additives as well, which may or may not be what you want.

Also, you have no idea how long ago that flour was milled or in what temperatures it has been stored. And finally, any microbes originally on the grain can't help you if they were killed off during processing by chemicals or high heat.

Instead of reaching for the cheapest or most convenient flour, take a look at what's beside it on those shelves. You might also look in your local natural foods store or co-op, or even just in the natural foods section of your supermarket. And check out the bulk bins, where flour may be fresher from faster turnover. With luck, you might find a store that keeps whole wheat flour refrigerated, or even a local mill that sells direct.

When choosing a brand, you can refer to package information, company reputation, the reviews or advice of other bakers, or what you find on the company's website. The final proof, though, is in the tasting. I've tried whole wheat flour of good repute that I simply would never use again. Choosing a different brand could make the difference between a dull-tasting sourdough and one you can hardly stop eating.

As to general *types* of whole wheat flour, you could use all-purpose whole wheat flour, or whole wheat bread flour, or about any type other than whole wheat pastry flour. Some blends of whole wheat *bread* flour, though, may sacrifice flavor to get their rising power—not a good trade-off, in my opinion. Again, the final test should be the taste.

Most whole wheat flour suited to bread is made from one or more kinds of hard "red" wheat, named after the reddish coloring caused by tannin in the bran. My own preference, though, is flour made from hard "white" wheat, which lacks that tannin. This absence translates to a sweeter taste and, to me and many other bakers, an improved one, without any loss of nutrition.

In the United States, flour from hard white wheat isn't as common as other kinds, but one brand often found in supermarkets is King Arthur White Whole Wheat Flour. That's what I've used for most of my recipe development and testing for this book. But I've also gotten great results from the regular King Arthur Whole Wheat Flour.

I should also warn you—just in case—to *not* use any flour made from *sprouted* wheat. Sprouting converts starches in the kernel to sugars, which will speed up fermenting and throw off the times in my recipes.

And now that I've talked about buying whole wheat flour, I'll tell you the honest truth: Unless you're buying direct from the mill, the very best whole wheat flour you can get is what you grind at home. But I don't want to slow you down from starting on your sourdough adventure, so I'll save that topic for a later chapter.

No matter what whole wheat flour you get or grind, make sure to refrigerate any of it not used within a day or so. Unlike white flour, whole wheat flour contains enough oil to go rancid, which turns it bitter. To keep moisture away from it in the refrigerator, you can transfer the flour to an airtight food storage container or just place the original bag inside a plastic one.

Using whole wheat flour in sourdough or any other bread does create one problem: The edges of the wheat bran cut the dough's gluten into smaller pieces. This results in a loaf with less rise than most people like, and it can also make for slices that fall apart, especially as the loaf dries out. So, for my basic recipe, I counterbalance the whole wheat with regular (white) unbleached bread flour—or *strong flour*, as it's called in the United Kingdom.

Choosing a bread flour can be tricky, because some can include additives that overstrengthen the gluten. Such additives are common in modern commercial baking, which may explain why so many people have recently found themselves "gluten sensitive."

For this book and my personal baking, I've mostly used King Arthur Unbleached Bread Flour. Note that this has a bit higher gluten content than the more common brands, and it also includes some malted barley flour for yeast (and bacteria) growth—but it does not seem to include the gluten strengtheners I try to avoid. For a real taste treat, try the organic version, King Arthur Organic Unbleached Bread Flour.

If using bread flour is inconvenient, or if you're worried about what's been added, you can use all-purpose instead. Most brands have enough gluten for bread, and in some cases, you might not even notice the difference. There are exceptions, though—especially among regional brands in the southern United States—so make sure you're getting a protein content of at least 9%. Personally, I've had good results from King Arthur Unbleached All-Purpose Flour, with its protein content of 11.7%.

Blending whole wheat flour with regular bread flour or all-purpose flour gives a decent compromise between nutrition and rise—but if you're in the United Kingdom or mainland Europe, you might try a different solution. Bakers there may have access to *high extraction* flour. That may sound like flour with more taken out, but it's the opposite.

Here's how it works: Most modern milling of wheat starts by extracting all bran and germ. (Milling by stone grinding is an exception.) At this point, it's just white flour. To then make whole wheat flour, bran and germ are *added*—supposedly, enough of each to match the amounts taken out. For high extraction flour, on the other hand, only a *high percentage* of the "extraction" is replaced—most but not all of the original amounts. The effect is much like blending white and whole wheat flours.

For a 24-hour sourdough with no starter, you're relying entirely on the bacteria content of your flour. That bacteria content can change not only among different brands and types of flour but even within the same type and brand. So, don't be shocked if opening a new bag gives you a somewhat different sourdough.

Water

Water quality is an obsession with home brewers, as it greatly affects their brews. But oddly, sourdough bakers seem to seldom give it much thought, though it affects their bread just as much.

Truthfully, tap water is *usually* fine for sourdough, but you should still be aware of problems that water can cause.

Water has two qualities that affect sourdough. One is the acid/alkaline balance, determined by the relative amounts of acids and alkalies dissolved in the water. The other is hardness/softness, based on the amount of minerals.

These qualities are separate but related. For instance, the minerals in "hard" water will *buffer* the acids in the water, turning it more alkaline. Conversely, "soft" water tends to be acid. In fact, if you remove *all* minerals from the water—as in water that's distilled or purified—it will quickly absorb carbon dioxide from the air and convert it to carbonic acid, tilting the balance even more. The mineral-free water in those supermarket bottles is far from neutral!

What does this have to do with sourdough? Sourdough microbes prefer an acid environment for their growth, with some preferring it *very* acid. Would it be best, then, to use distilled or filtered water? No, because there's another factor: Gluten needs minerals to develop strength—chiefly calcium and magnesium. If you use distilled or filtered water, you're weakening your gluten and limiting your rise.

After trying or considering a number of options—buying different bottled waters, adding minerals, even replacing water with bottled apple juice (which turned out particularly badly, producing a foul, bitter taste)—I decided that my tap water worked well enough. But if you find your water excessively hard or soft, one simple fix is to use bottled spring water instead. This will supply minerals but without being too hard or too alkaline.

If you're not sure about your own tap water, you should be able to get information from your local water utility. You can also test the acid/alkaline balance of your water and other liquids with a digital pH meter. (More on that in the chapter "Testing Your Sourdough.")

There's another water quality issue, which sourdough bakers *do* sometimes think of: chlorine content. That's the stuff put in tap water to kill microbes—all kinds, including the kinds we're trying to nurture. Personally, I've never noticed any effect of chlorine on my sourdough—but on the other hand, it doesn't make much sense to me to add something with a chance of causing harm.

Luckily, there's a simple solution to this problem: keep a pitcher of water on your kitchen counter. The chlorine evaporates from the water within a day or two, so you know it's safe to use—and as a bonus, the water is conveniently at room temperature when you're ready to make the sponge. But if you can't wait a day or two and your chlorine problem is serious enough, you could instead boil your water for about twenty minutes.

These methods won't work, though, if your water utility uses *chloramines*—chlorine combined with ammonia—instead of straight chlorine. One method that will work on chlorine *or* chloramines is to add a pinch of ascorbic acid to a pitcher of water. (Technically, a pinch is 1⁄16 teaspoon, if you want to measure it.) Amazingly, this *instantly* rids it of all chlorine, as I've verified with a "free chlorine" test strip. Also said to work are a few drops of lemon juice—or basically, any liquid or powdered source of vitamin C. In such tiny amounts, it shouldn't hurt your bread and might even help—but of course, you'll want to test that.

Home water filters may or may not help with chlorine and chloramines. To find one that will, look for a filter with "granular activated charcoal," "carbon block filtration," "briquette filtration," or "membrane filtration" (reverse osmosis).

Or if chlorine is a serious problem, again, you can use bottled spring water.

Salt

My advice is to use whatever cheap, common table salt you have on hand. That's what I've done, and it's what my teaspoon measurements are based on. Many people, though, will try to make the choice more complicated for you, advocating exotic salts that really have no advantage.

You see, if salt is to be sold commercially, it must by law be crystallized. And for salt to crystallize, it must first be almost completely pure—in other words, nearly 100% sodium chloride. That means there are no significant extra nutrients in any kind of salt you can buy, regardless of description or marketing hype.

If you see color in salt, it's *not* from minerals within the crystals—it's from something they're mixed together with. Take for example the many gourmet sea salts from around the world, which are made in low-tech evaporation ponds. Their color is generally due to a residue of clay and algae from the ponds themselves—in other words, mud and sludge. Sometimes clay or ground rock is added purposely as well. (None of this is great for your tooth enamel!)

Mined salts too can have color—such as the pink of the wildly popular but falsely named Himalayan salt (actually mined south of there in the hills of prosaic Pakistan). Here again, the color comes only from mixed-in impurities that provide no practical benefit.

An interesting factoid: In the United States, big companies legally can and do sell the exact same salt as both regular table salt and sea salt. That's because, whether taken from the sea or from a mine, it *all* originally came from the sea. And once it's processed commercially, it's identical anyway.

What *can* differ in the crystals of specialty salts is the structure. Some salt crystals are more irregular than others, and those with more surface area will impart a stronger taste when contacting your tongue. If you're sprinkling such salt on dry food, you can get the same saltiness with less salt. But when measuring by volume, that same irregular structure keeps the salt from packing as tightly—so to compensate, you need to use *more*. That's because, once the salt is dissolved—as in sourdough—*any difference in structure or taste vanishes entirely.*

If you want to read more about salt myths and scams, I highly recommend *What Einstein Told His Cook*, by Robert L. Wolke.

Some bakers recommend against iodized salt for its taste. I won't argue with them, but I personally don't notice the difference. And having a sister with a history of hyperthyroidism, I'm a firm believer in using salt that's iodized. In any case, the tiny amount doesn't seem to hurt the growth of the sourdough bacteria, as far as I can tell.

Yeast

The two types of yeast most often found in markets are *active dry* and *instant*, both in the form of dry granules. The granules of active dry yeast are larger, with a coating of dead yeast cells around a core of live ones. You need heat and moisture to break through the coating and revive the live yeast, and that's normally done by stirring the yeast into warm water ahead of time. In my recipes, though, the yeast is added to the dough when it's both wet and warm, so you do *not* need to activate the yeast separately.

Another issue with active dry yeast is that the dead cells that coat the granules can contribute an undesirable taste to bread. But so little yeast is added in my recipes—just ⅛ teaspoon in my basic recipe, ¼ teaspoon in some others—that this really doesn't matter. After all, it's only the live yeast that multiply, not the dead ones!

Instant yeast—also called *rapid-rise*—will also work in my recipes. In fact, with its smaller, uncoated granules for adding directly to dough, it should theoretically work more quickly and reliably—but in practice, I've found no difference.

At the same time, instant yeast can include the same kind of questionable gluten strengtheners you sometimes find in bread flour. For safety and predictability, then, I prefer active dry—though, here again, the amount of yeast in my recipes is so small, any additives should have little effect on the bread.

Don't make the mistake of assuming you can use yeast right up to its expiration, or "best by," date. That date is meant only for an *unopened* jar. Once the jar is open, the yeast deteriorates much more quickly. Even when refrigerated, it's supposed to be used in the next four months.

You can stretch its useful life by doubling your yeast measurements or more. Even so, with the tiny amounts used in smart sourdough, you might wind up throwing out some or even most of the yeast—but that's better than stressing over bread taking forever to rise.

Flour Fallacies

We've already looked at a number of myths surrounding sourdough. Here are a few just about flour. (My thanks for some of the information on bran goes to William Alexander and his thoroughly enjoyable book *52 Loaves*.)

Myth: Traditionally, most wheat flour was 100% whole wheat.

Not really. In a traditional flour mill, the grinding stones took bran off the kernels in flakes and flattened the germ. The largest pieces were then removed by sifting. So, most traditional wheat flour was closer to what's available today in the United Kingdom and the rest of Europe as *high extraction* flour, with somewhat less bran and germ than it started with. In the United States, we can get something similar by blending whole wheat flour and regular bread flour, as I do in my basic recipe.

Myth: Mixing unbleached bread flour into whole wheat helps the dough rise by increasing gluten.

It helps the dough rise mostly by reducing the relative amount of bran, as bran will cut the gluten strands. It *may* also increase gluten—but depending on the flour, it could do the opposite! For example, King Arthur's regular whole wheat flour has a gluten content of 14.0% and its white whole wheat flour has 13.0%, while its unbleached bread flour has only 12.7%. So, mixing the bread flour with either of the whole wheat flours will *reduce* its gluten—though not enough to worry about.

Myth: For a better rise, you can make high extraction flour from whole wheat by sifting out some bran.

That's the advice you commonly read, and there are home flour sifters sold just for that purpose. But this really depends on the kind of wheat and how it was milled.

With roller milling, bran is completely removed in large pieces before being added back for whole wheat flour, and much of this bran can be sifted out later. But impact mills shatter the bran into tiny bits, and grinding stones do the same to bran of the harder strains of wheat common today. Most of these bits are no larger than other flour particles, making them impossible to remove.

So, for example, if you run King Arthur White Whole Wheat Flour through a 40-mesh flour sifter, it won't remove much bran at all, and it *won't* improve your rise. (Yes, I've tried it.)

Myth: Stone-ground flour is always superior.

Stone grinding is often used by companies that take pride in their product—but by itself, it doesn't guarantee high quality. The most tasteless commercial whole wheat flour I've ever tried was labeled stone ground.

Part of this depends on how the mill is operated. Any commercial mill can be run hard and fast enough to cook the flour—and then it won't matter what kind of mill it is. By the same token, any mill can be run more slowly for lower heat and a superior product.

Stone-ground flour, though, does have one indisputable advantage. With most other milling, bran and germ are first separated from the rest of the wheat kernel—then, if whole wheat flour is desired, they're added back at the end. The amounts replaced are *supposed* to be about the same as the amounts removed. But at least in the United States, that's not legally required, and the companies themselves seldom tell you what they're doing. So, you usually have no way to be sure of the flour's true content.

With stone grinding, on the other hand, bran and germ are generally *not* separated out—and in fact, with most modern wheat strains, they *can't* be to any great extent. So, you're much more sure to be getting all or nearly all of the kernel.

The Right Equipment

Let's take a look at the equipment you'll need for smart sourdough. Note that some of these items are more essential than others. For some you don't have, you might find workable substitutes in your kitchen.

Warming Device

The most important piece of equipment you'll need is a warming device. For my recipes, this device must be able to heat water to a range around 100°F (around 38°C) and keep it there, with no swings larger than a degree or two in either direction.

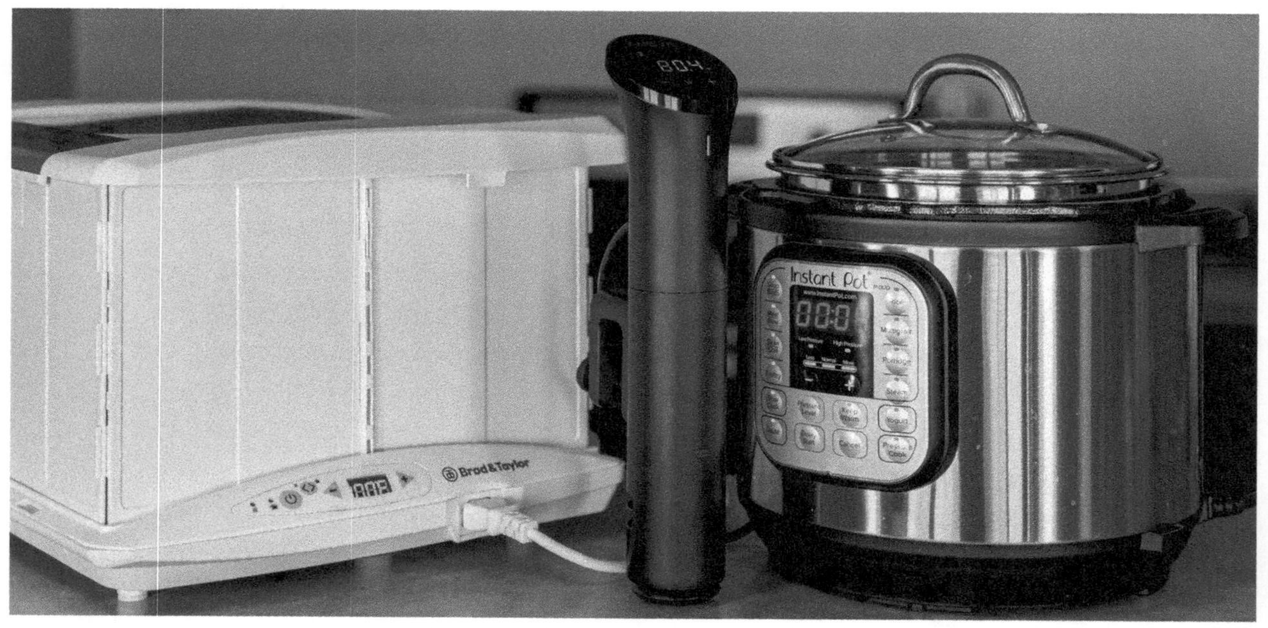

Warming devices for smart sourdough

(Since sourdough generates its own, inconstant heat, it's best to use water to test your device and adjust its setup.)

Getting to the right temperature range might be trickier than you'd expect, because this is a range that most warming devices avoid as unsafe for most food. With meat, for example, one of the last things you want is to encourage the growth of bacteria—but that's *exactly* what you want to do with sourdough. So, you may have to tinker with your device's setup to get it to heat in the right range.

With a little ingenuity and flexibility, a number of warming devices can be adapted for smart sourdough, and I'll point the way in the chapter "The Right Setup." I'll also give detailed instructions for several devices, including the Instant Pot (used as a slow cooker) and a sous vide cooker.

Still, for combined accuracy, flexibility, convenience, and roominess, I believe the home baker has one best choice: the Brød & Taylor Folding Proofer & Slow Cooker. It's a clever and innovative contraption introduced only in 2011—a simple plastic box with a heating element under a metal floor.

Place your food container directly on that floor, and it's a slow cooker—but place it on a rack *above* that floor, and you get a proofer with a range of 70°F to 120°F (21°C to 49°C). What's more, the Proofer Mode uses not direct heating but radiant heating, which works much better for sourdough at high temperatures. (More on that too in the chapter on setup.)

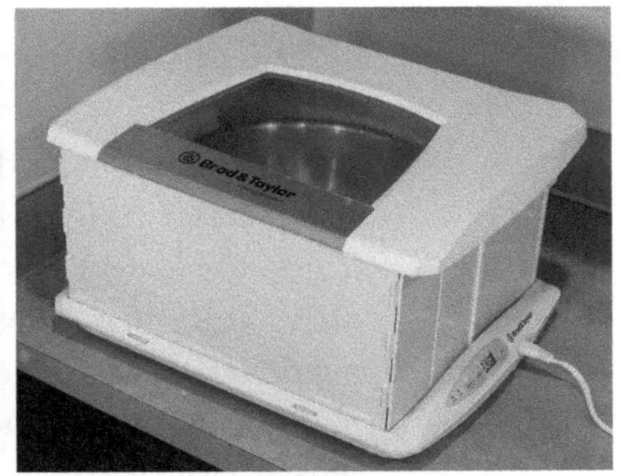

Brød & Taylor Folding Proofer

The proofer is large enough to hold a big mixing bowl or two large loaf pans, yet folds down flat when not in use. It even includes a water tray to produce steam for humidity while your loaf is rising.

To possibly save you time, I'll also mention one type of device that does *not* work well for smart sourdough: a kitchen or countertop oven. Because ovens are designed mainly for *much* higher temperatures, they have much more powerful heating elements. So, even when an oven can be set to a temperature low enough for sourdough—which is rare—it can't hold it there steadily enough. At the same time, the old trick of heating with the oven's pilot light alone will *not* raise the temperature to the range we want.

Other Equipment

Here's the rest of what you'll need for my basic recipe. Some of these items are needed only with specific warming devices, and I'll talk more about their use in the chapter on setup.

Kitchen scale. For reasons explained in the sidebar "Why Weigh Your Flour?", all my flour measurements in this book are by weight. So, you'll definitely need a decent scale.

Your scale should be digital and should display weight in tenths of an ounce. (That's easier to work with than grams and plenty precise enough for sourdough.) It should also have a tare button so you can reset the weight to zero after placing a new container on the scale. (But if yours doesn't have that button, you can instead turn the scale off and on again after placing the container.)

Avoid scales with the display facing straight up—as it does on many cheaper models. If you place a large bowl on one of these scales, the bowl will cover the display! But if you already have such a scale, here's a workaround: Place a jar or small plastic tub facedown on the scale, then balance your bowl on top of that.

Folding thermometer. A decent thermometer is nearly indispensable for smart sourdough. This is not only to tell if your bread is done baking but also to check on your sourdough's temperature

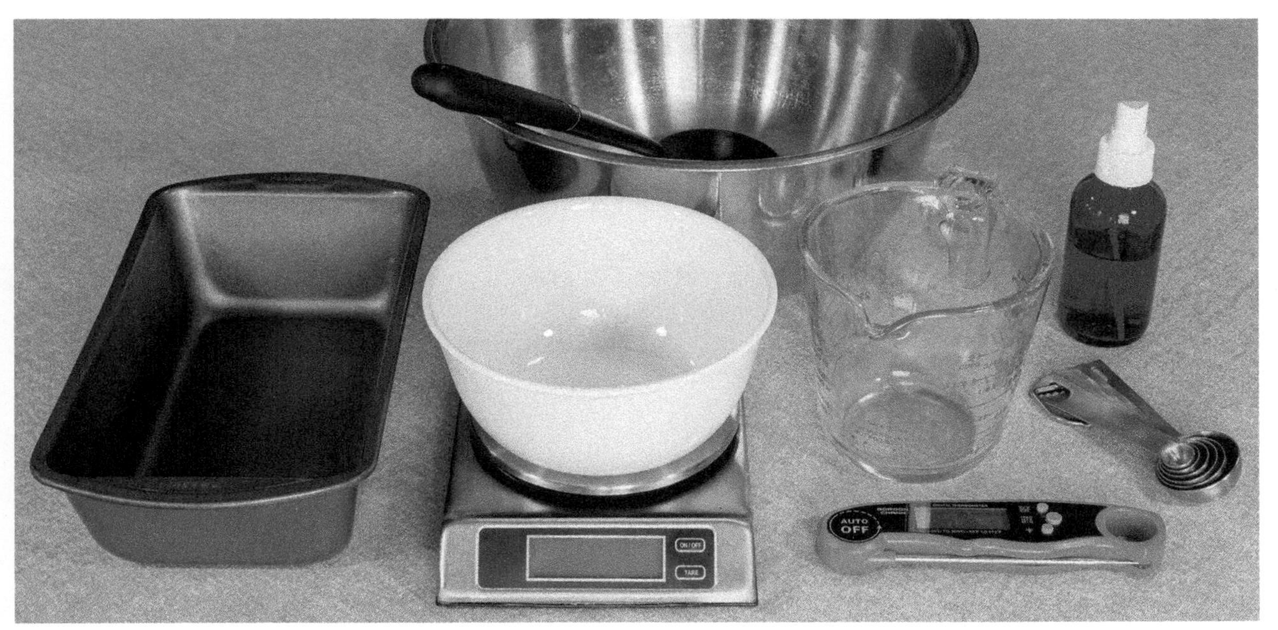

Other equipment for smart sourdough

while fermenting—not to mention testing your warming device before actually making sourdough.

Because a sourdough sponge is so shallow, it really requires the short, angled stem of a folding thermometer. The original and best known of these is the Thermapen, but many cheaper, adequate imitations are now available.

Don't be confused by the multitude of such imitations sold online. They are probably almost all made in one or two factories in China but slightly customized for small companies to sell under their own brand names. That means the complaints you read about some will apply to most others, even if the companies have managed to stuff or falsify their reviews. That's not to say you can't use the thermometers, but don't bother spending much time choosing one over the other.

Whatever the quality of your thermometer, it's a good idea to test it when you get it and occasionally after that. The best way to test is to compare the thermometer's reading to a known temperature. Typically, this is the temperature of an ice bath—32°F (0°C)—or of boiling water—nominally 212°F (100°C), but varying by altitude above sea level, atmospheric pressure, and other factors. Details for testing can easily be found online.

Thermometers that are off by a degree or two Fahrenheit (one degree Celsius) are still considered okay. But even for a larger error, you can just mentally add or subtract the difference when reading the temperature of your sourdough.

Mixing bowl. You'll need a mixing bowl large enough to hold your sourdough, and hopefully large enough to contain the mess you make when mixing flour and water. In fact, if you take my later advice, you'll want it large enough to allow kneading by hand, right in the bowl!

My favorite is a six-quart stainless steel bowl, slightly under a foot wide to fit nicely in my Brød & Taylor proofer. If the setup for your warming device requires something smaller, a four-quart bowl also does well.

Because of the acids produced by sourdough, this bowl needs to be reasonably nonreactive. Good kinds can include stainless steel, ceramic, and glass. Be cautious, though, about cheap bowls made in countries where manufacturing standards are lax.

The bowl also needs to conduct heat fairly well. That means *no silicone or other plastic*—not even for the base alone, as with stainless steel bowls called "non-slip" or "non-skid." Since you'll most likely be heating from below with radiant heat, a plastic bowl or base can lower your temperatures drastically.

Kitchen spoon. The spoon you use to stir the sponge and mix the dough should be big enough and sturdy enough for this heavy job. It should also be able to resist mild acid, just like your mixing bowl.

I like to use a wooden spoon, the bulkiest I can find—partly because I just like its feel in my hand. But a stainless steel or plastic spoon can do well, too, with less chance of discoloring over time.

Loaf pan. My basic instructions are for a sandwich loaf, so you'll need a loaf pan to follow them exactly. (I'll discuss round loaves later, in the chapter "Baking in the Round.")

Bread loaf pans come in large, medium, and small sizes. In the past, the medium was considered "standard," but with today's preference for airy bread, only the large is still common—so that's what my main recipes use, even though my sourdough is decidedly *not* airy. But in case you own a medium or small pan or just prefer a smaller loaf, I offer recipe variations for those sizes in the chapter "Scaling Your Sourdough."

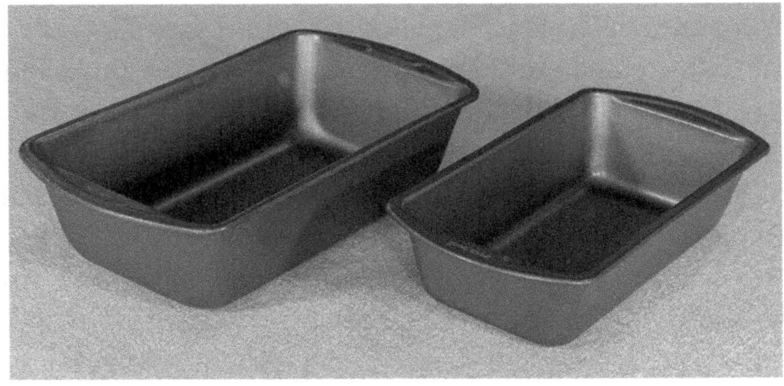

Large and medium ("standard") loaf pans

Not sure which size pan you have? Measurements given for loaf pans tend to be nominal rather than real, but the Loaf Pan Sizes chart should tell you enough to recognize your pan by its actual measurements or by how it's described. Note that the chart's lengths and widths measure the opening at the *top* of the pan, as is customary. (In product descriptions, some vendors

Loaf Pan Sizes

	LARGE	MEDIUM	SMALL
Nominal loaf weight (pounds)	1½ or 2	1	¾
Nominal volume (cups)	8	6	4
Typical dimensions (inches)	9 × 5 × 3	8½ × 4½ × 2½	8 × 4 × 2½
Typical dimensions (centimeters)	23 × 13 × 8	21 × 11 × 6	20 × 10 × 6

may unhelpfully measure at the bottom instead, which can make a pan sound like the next size down. Others may include the pan's handles in the length, making it sound larger.)

As with your bowls, your loaf pan can be made of any material that resists acid and conducts heat well. In other words, *do not use silicone*. A nonstick coating is good, though you'll likely *still* need to oil or grease the pan lightly. (Or you could use parchment paper, as my wife does.)

Most loaf pans today are "seamless," stamped from a single piece of metal. I like them, because they're easier to clean and are most likely to have handles, which can make it much easier and safer to get the loaf out. In the large size, though, they do have one disadvantage: For easier manufacturing, they're designed shorter and wider than traditional loaf pans, yielding a squatter loaf.

At least as important as material and form is *color*. Dark pans cook the crust better, making it pull away from the pan so the loaf most often just falls out. Getting a loaf out of a light-colored pan—even a "nonstick" one—can be a real chore. Dark loaf pans, then, are the only kind I recommend. My own favorites are the dark nonstick pans from GoodCook.

Plastic dishpan or other water container (for sous vide). You'll need a water container deep enough for your sous vide cooker and wide enough to float your mixing bowl. A rectangular shape rather than square may be best for fitting both cooker and bowl.

Wire rack (for slow cooker or sous vide). As I'll explain in detail in the chapter on setup, a wire rack provides a simple way to convert a direct heat device like an Instant Pot or other slow cooker into a lower-temperature device with radiant heating. And it can do the same for sous vide, so you can warm your loaf pan without setting it in the water. A cooling rack works well for these purposes.

Cake cover or other cover (for slow cooker or sous vide). This is used along with your wire rack to collect steam while the loaf is rising—again, as I explain in the chapter on setup. The cake cover you get should be clear plastic, so you can see inside. Also make sure it's wide enough for your pan! My cover is nominally twelve-inch, but the opening at the bottom measures 11½ inches—and for my loaf pan, that's a fairly tight fit.

Of course, you can improvise a different cover, but try to make it transparent.

Flour sack towel (optional). This is a light, loose-weave, plain white cotton kitchen towel. Don't confuse it with a tea towel—a linen towel that's likely to be dyed.

This towel is one of those things you *might* be able to do without but that you're likely to be glad to have on hand. It's ideal, for instance, for covering your mixing bowl to protect your sourdough from dust or insects—especially while it's being warmed. Unlike solid covers, it will never cause moisture to condense and drip back onto your sourdough. And if your setup doesn't provide steam to prevent your loaves from crusting, a towel placed over the pan can at least slow it down.

To keep the towel from dipping into your mixing bowl, tuck the ends underneath.

Mister (optional). A mister is a small spray bottle with a fine spray, and it's another item you'll likely be glad to have. If steam isn't stopping your loaf from crusting, you can spritz water on it to slow the crusting or even partially reverse it.

Bowl scraper (optional). This is a flat piece of plastic with a curved edge. It can be used to clean mixing bowls or unglazed stoneware after soaking. I've also found it handy for dividing dough from large recipes to make smaller loaves.

Plastic bags (optional). I like to store my bread in plastic bags, but the gallon-size bags sold in the supermarket aren't quite big enough. So, I buy clear bread or grocery bags, 12 inches by 20 inches, which come in a roll. There are many brands—the ones I buy are from Decony.

Other. Of course, you'll use other equipment you're likely to have already in your kitchen: smaller bowls, knives, measuring cups and spoons, a cooling rack (for actual cooling), pot holders or oven mitts, a timer. Oh, and an oven for baking.

You may notice that this list is missing a stand mixer or food processor. I don't recommend them, as I consider kneading by hand to be better suited to sourdough in general and my recipes in particular. (More details on that later, in the sidebar "The Joy of Kneading.") On the other hand, if you're set on using one—or if you *must*, because of a physical condition—it certainly won't stop you from making good sourdough.

Why Weigh Your Flour?

If you've read many books on baking, you've probably already run into exhortations to weigh your flour—and then found that the book still humored you by measuring in cups as well.

When I started this book, I too planned to offer both measurements—until I realized how meaningless the cup measurement can be. The amount of flour in a cup can vary according to the type of flour, the brand, and maybe most importantly, how you handle the flour during measuring.

As an extreme case, here's the comparison I made for myself of two different flours I used in testing (with the numbers slightly rounded). King Arthur White Whole Wheat Flour, scooped from the bag and dropped into a liquid measuring cup, was almost 6 ounces per cup. But flour I ground at home from white wheat berries and scooped up with the same measuring cup was only 4½ ounces per cup—three-quarters as much!

Though there is a standard way of measuring flour to even out such differences, the truth is that you can't count on anyone using it—partly because they may not know, and partly because it's too much trouble anyway. So, the only way a cooking writer can ensure accuracy and consistency is with measurements by weight.

Another problem I ran into with cup measurements was in working out my recipe variations, which are based on percentages. I didn't think my readers would appreciate weird fractional amounts like 75% of 1½ cups.

In case your calculator isn't handy, that's 1⅛ cups—and a standard cup cannot measure in eighths!

The Right Conditions

A big part of making sourdough is setting up conditions so sourdough microbes can thrive. Knowing about these conditions will help you understand the method behind smart sourdough—and also help you adjust it, if needed.

Here are the factors we need to look at:

- Temperature—how warm you keep your sourdough
- Hydration—the proportion of water in it
- Acidity—the level of acid
- Salinity—the proportion of salt
- Aeration—the amount of air mixed in
- Humidity—the moistness of the surrounding air

Temperature

There's no factor more important in making sourdough than temperature. And greater *control* of this factor is the biggest difference between traditional sourdough methods and smart sourdough.

For most home sourdough bakers, temperature control doesn't go much beyond placing sourdough in a "warm spot" in their home or at times in a refrigerator to "retard" it. This rough approach has led to some fanciful ideas, such as that sourdough bacteria are more active at lower temperatures.

Actually, the opposite is true. Sourdough bacteria are most active at well above room temperature. But in their optimum range, those bacteria produce much less acetic acid and much more lactic acid, which tastes and smells less sour. If you lower the temperature, on the other hand, it stresses the bacteria, the proportion of acetic acid increases, and with it the sour taste and smell. So, the bacteria *seem* to be more active, even while they're less so.

Some sourdough bakers have learned better from a widely shared 1998 scientific study on sourdough cultures from the University of Hohenheim in Germany, conducted by Michael G. Gänzle and colleagues. But generalizing about its results has led to a *different* misconception—that peak growth of sourdough bacteria occurs right at 32°C to 33°C (90°F to 91°F).

What gets mostly overlooked is that this study was for only one species of sourdough bacteria—*Lactobacillus sanfranciscensis*, named for its importance in San Francisco sourdough but actually found worldwide. It is often dominant in sourdough starters developed at room temperature or slightly higher. But sourdough normally includes many other species of lactic acid bacteria as well.

For many of these other bacteria, the optimum temperature is higher. In fact, the bacteria called *thermophilic* ("heat loving") don't hit their stride till around 113°F (45°C)—a temperature already too high for *L. sanfranciscensis* and some other species. That temperature is used for some Type II sourdough, which is typically inoculated with commercial culture made from isolated thermophilic species. (The same temperature is common for yogurt making, since store-bought yogurt too is made with commercial cultures.)

As the temperature of sourdough goes up, different species gain the advantage and can achieve dominance. A difference of just a few degrees can completely change the "species profile" of the sourdough, and with it, the taste. But that's not the only effect. Higher temperatures also speed up the fermenting—

Sourdough Temperature

Faster fermenting
More lactic acid
Favors bacteria over yeast
Favors heat-loving bacteria
Favors gas production over yeast growth
Greater risk of runaway activity

Slower fermenting
More acetic acid
Favors yeast over bacteria
Favors non-heat-loving bacteria
Favors yeast growth over gas production
Less risk of runaway activity

and at some point can increase the risk of runaway microbe activity.

How, then, to choose the best temperature for smart sourdough? To start with, it should be within the range of 90°F to 110°F (32°C to 43°C). That range starts where sourdough bacteria start to outpace most sourdough yeast, and it ends just short of where some species of sourdough bacteria start to weaken and die.

Having tried several temperatures in that range, I've settled on 105°F (about 40°C) as the optimum sourdough temperature for a 24-hour recipe. This seems to provide the best balance of fermenting speed and manageability. It also supports an especially wide variety of sourdough bacteria species. Maybe that's why my smart sourdough is so rich in flavor!

Note, though, that this is *not* meant as a *constant* temperature for the sourdough. As I'll discuss further in the chapter "The Right Method," heat is generated by the ever-changing microbe activity in the sourdough itself. As this heat increases and decreases, it can make the sourdough temperature fluctuate by several degrees in either direction. So, the optimum temperature I've cited is actually more of a midpoint, with real temperatures ranging above and below.

Note too that this is *not* a setting for your warming device. To figure that setting, you'll need to factor in the way you're using the device and also the heat added by the sourdough. But I'll discuss all that in the chapter "The Right Setup."

So far, I've talked only about temperatures for the sourdough *bacteria*. And in the early stages of smart sourdough, that's pretty much all you need to deal with. Even in a traditional starter, yeast is scarce at first, showing up in significant amounts only after the first few days and feeding cycles. And in *smart* sourdough, the bacteria's initial dominance is actually boosted, because high temperature favors them over the yeast.

But things change when you add baker's yeast—which you do in my method at the end, when you make the loaf. Baker's yeast itself has a very specific optimum temperature—well, actually, two of them. Its optimum temperature for *growth* is 90°F (32°C). But its optimum temperature for producing gas to make your bread rise is a little higher—95°F (35°C).

It's this second optimum that interests us, as we want to make the bread rise with *minimal* yeast growth. This helps us reduce alcohol in the bread, since alcohol can overpower the wonderful sourdough tastes we're trying to develop.

But hold on, there's a problem. For the rising loaf, we now have *two* optimum temperatures to consider: one for the bacteria, and a lower one for the added yeast. My solution is simply to split the difference. As the optimum temperature for my loaf—after the yeast and final flour are added—I've settled on 100°F (38°C).

Hydration, Aeration, and Humidity

Hydration is a fancy name for the amount of water in your sourdough, relative to the amount of flour. Microbes multiply more readily when there's plenty of water. Also, at high hydration, the sourdough bacteria produce an even higher proportion of lactic acid relative to acetic acid, giving a milder taste and smell. With lower hydration—less water, relatively—you get less growth but more sourness.

With smart sourdough, we take advantage of these facts by starting with a highly hydrated *sponge*—or, to be specific, we start by mixing all of the recipe water with only some of the flour. This maximizes bacteria growth at the beginning. Then, as we feed the sponge with more flour and finally make the loaf, we have more bacteria on hand for souring.

Sourdough bacteria are mostly *anaerobic*—meaning, they do best when there's no oxygen around. Many less desirable microbes, on the other hand, are *aerobic*—preferring to have oxygen—or can go either way.

This means, for one thing, that you want to avoid beating too much air into your sourdough sponge—something that's easy to do with mechanical mixing. But even when sourdough

Sourdough Hydration

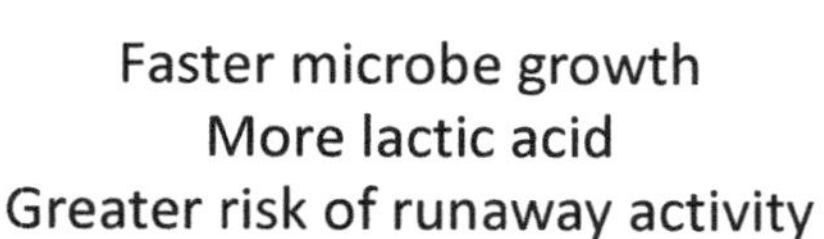

Slower microbe growth
More acetic acid
Less risk of runaway activity

Sourdough Aeration

Inhibits bacteria
Boosts undesirable microbes

Boosts bacteria
Inhibits undesirable microbes

bacteria are developing nicely within the sponge in the absence of much air, you can still get undesirable microbes growing on the sponge's surface, where air is plentiful. This unwanted growth becomes *more* likely at higher temperatures, and it's a special problem when there's high humidity, which these microbes love.

The surface microbes can include mold but also yeast, which in smart sourdough we want to suppress at first. This surface yeast even has a special name among home fermenters, who call it "Kahm yeast" and likewise consider it a nuisance. Given the relatively short fermenting times in breadmaking, the chances of growing any really harmful microbes on a sponge are almost nil—but surface microbes can still spoil the taste of your bread.

How to handle this? Though it's hard to keep air from the surface of a sponge, we *can* reduce humidity. So, for a sponge with raised temperature, it's best not to cover it in any way that traps moisture. Generally, that means using dry cloth instead of a dish, plastic wrap, or anything else more solid or less permeable—that is, if you need a cover at all.

Keeping the air dry also allows the sponge surface to crust over, more or less, which reduces moisture for surface microbes and also stops air from migrating into the sponge. That helps keep the sponge healthy for long enough to get decently sour. Of course, to keep the crusting, you'll want to avoid stirring the sponge unless it's time to add ingredients.

Acidity

The benefits of sourdough mostly come from the lactic and acetic acids that sourdough bacteria produce. But these acids don't benefit just you—to a point, they benefit the bacteria too! The acids create an environment in which the sourdough bacteria themselves are more comfortable. And that's partly because those same acids discourage or even kill most competing microbes.

Just as different species of sourdough bacteria thrive best at different temperatures, they also thrive best at different levels of acidity. This is a good part of what traditional sourdough starters and smart sourdough are both about: gradually stepping up the acidity to favor the microbes that produce the most acid and also thrive on it the most. (I'll discuss that in the chapter on method.)

I said the acids help *to a point*, because sourdough can collect so much acid that even the sourdough bacteria are suppressed or killed. But within the short time frame of smart sourdough, we don't have to worry about that.

A side effect of the higher acidity is that it strengthens the gluten, enabling a higher rise. In doing that, lactic and acetic acids are the natural substitutes for the ascorbic acid often added to bread today as a dough conditioner. (Adding ascorbic acid is one of the tricks of "rapid-rise" yeast.)

Sourdough Acidity

Favors acid-loving bacteria and yeast
Inhibits undesirable microbes
Strengthens gluten

Favors non-acid-loving bacteria and yeast
Allows undesirable microbes

Sourdough Salinity

Inhibits all microbe growth
Favors sourdough bacteria and yeast

Allows all microbe growth

Salinity

As I pointed out before, one of the myths about sourdough is that salt discourages the growth of sourdough bacteria. Now, it's true that salt inhibits the growth of these microbes—but only by about 10%, according to one study. And that was measured in a culture where such microbes were isolated, growing without competition from other species.

Meanwhile, the same salt inhibits the growth of undesirable, *competing* organisms *even more*. So, adding salt early actually gives the sourdough microbes a leg up, reducing the time they need to reach dominance—as well as reducing the chance of something else entirely taking over.

It *is* possible to add too much salt, which could kill the microbes. But as long as you're adding only enough for taste, you'll be well within limits.

Other Conditions

Are there any other conditions affecting sourdough? Probably. As baker/microbiologist Debra Wink likes to say, "It's never that simple with living things."

So, when you get up in the morning, be careful not to look at your sourdough funny, or it might come out completely different. And for heaven's sake, keep it out of the light of a full moon!

The Right Method

It's often said that fermenting dough properly takes time. But what it really takes is *activity*. If chemical reactions and the functions of bacteria are sped up, less time is needed.

With smart sourdough, we manipulate conditions to do exactly that, fitting the development of our sourdough into 24 hours or less. Not that you can strictly copy the development of a sourdough starter in that time—but you can come close enough to produce a healthful and wonderfully tangy loaf of bread, aided only by a little baker's yeast for the rise.

Let's see how that works.

Cycles of Sourness

When you mix flour and water, you get an active soup of flour, microbes, and the enzymes that break down the flour's starch into sugar that the microbes can eat.

Among these microbes are *lactic acid bacteria*. When these bacteria eat the sugar made available to them, they release waste products that include lactic acid and acetic acid. These two acids supply most of the taste associated with sourdough, along with its health benefits. Lactic acid gives a sourness like that of yogurt, while acetic acid gives a sourness like that of vinegar. Ideally, your sourdough will have a nice blend of both tastes.

One effect of these acids is to inhibit microbe growth—even the growth of the lactic acid bacteria themselves. But those bacteria, along with some species of yeast, are *less* affected by the acid than other microbes are. So, the acid gives them an advantage in staying active, helping them to grab a larger share of sugar and use it to multiply throughout the sourdough.

When bakers make a traditional sourdough starter, a mixture of flour and water is given a series of "feedings" over several days. For each feeding, some of the starter is removed, and more flour and water are added. This supplies more starch to break down into sugar and also dilutes and buffers the acid, giving the microbes a renewed chance for growth.

But despite the dilution, the starter begins each new cycle with a little more acid than it had at the start of the previous one. So, the cycles increasingly favor bacteria and yeast that tolerate that acid.

Of course, these are also the bacteria that *produce* the most acid. So, the starter winds up with a collection of microbes that produce a lot of acid *and* are especially tolerant of it—and that's the goal. To *maintain* the starter at that point, it's fed less frequently and often stored at a lower temperature.

Just as with a traditional starter, smart sourdough builds sourness with a succession of feeding cycles. But there are several crucial differences.

- The cycles are sped up, mainly by raising temperature, to fit several cycles into 24 hours.
- Feedings are calculated so no sourdough is *ever* removed and discarded. It all goes into the loaf you're making!
- The sourdough is started from scratch for each baking, which takes place within a day—so there is *zero* maintenance between times you make bread.

Phases of Feeding

The main trick in developing sourdough—especially smart sourdough, with its compressed timing—is knowing when to feed it. So, let's take a close look at what happens in an individual feeding cycle. (I've gratefully drawn from a similar summary of "growth curve phases" by Kurt Janz.)

Adjustment phase. Each cycle starts with a period of low activity, when the microbes are adjusting to changes in their environment, and the enzymes are just starting to convert starch to sugar for the microbes to feed on.

Growth phase. Fueled by the available sugar, the microbes start multiplying. If temperature and other conditions are right, their growth accelerates rapidly, until the population is doubling or more every hour. The temperature of the sourdough rises a few degrees—about five degrees Fahrenheit (almost three degrees Celsius)—just from the biological activity of the microbes. Plentiful food and good conditions also mean that the lactic acid bacteria produce mostly lactic acid, with little or no acetic.

Plateau phase. Obviously, this rapid growth can't go on forever. Sooner or later, the exploding population of microbes starts to outpace the sugar supply. When this happens, growth of the microbes slows down and some microbes die, causing the population to level off. Temperature too stays steady.

Meanwhile, some lactic acid bacteria adopt different feeding patterns, causing them to produce acetic acid as well as lactic. Acetic acid has a fairly strong smell, while lactic acid has very little. So, it's only at this point, when the population has stabilized, that the sourdough starts to smell sour.

Stress phase. Even with a stable population, the microbes reach the point of struggling to survive on their share of available sugar. The growth rate drops, the death rate rises. Microbes start chewing through gluten as a last resort. Temperature slowly goes up another few degrees. Most important for the baker, lactic acid bacteria start producing much more acetic acid.

Ideally, it's sometime during this phase that you want to end your feeding cycle and start a new one. Though you may lose some gluten and there's some risk of sliding into the more destructive phase that follows, this is the phase in which your sourdough gains the most sour taste and smell.

Exhaustion phase. As food starts to run out, more and more microbes die off. The temperature spikes even higher—in some cases, enough to kill off more microbes. Feeding patterns of some lactic acid bacteria shift again. Instead of lactic and acetic acid, they produce mostly alcohol—a sourness *killer*—and carbon dioxide, a gas. In other words, they start producing mostly the same kind of waste as yeast.

In a sourdough starter or sponge, you can actually see when this is happening. On its surface, the sourdough starts fizzing or bubbling heavily, or "doming" as the crust lifts up. On stirring, you may find no gluten remaining at all, but only a runny mess that will give you dense, heavy bread.

Many traditional sourdough bakers mistake this surface activity as a sign that sourdough yeast are active, and they believe it means their starter is working. But in the early days of a starter, there's not enough yeast to produce such bubbling. Instead, it's the bacteria, and it means they're a short way from shutting down entirely.

Death phase. If the feeding cycle is allowed to continue—especially at high temperature—the last microbes starve, succumb to their own waste, and die. The sourdough stops generating much heat, and the temperature drops back toward where it started. Enzymes attack the dead microbes, and they stink as they decompose.

Feeding Cycle Phases

	Activity	Temperature gain	By-products
ADJUSTMENT	Low	Minimal	Minimal
GROWTH	Rising to high	Up to 5°F (3°C)	Mostly lactic acid
PLATEAU	High	5°F (3°C)	Lactic acid, some acetic
STRESS	High	Up to 10°F (6°C)	Acetic acid, some lactic
EXHAUSTION	High	Over 10°F (6°C)	Alcohol, carbon dioxide
DEATH	Low	Minimal	Minimal

You may recognize that strong, cheesy smell, if you've ever eaten nutritional yeast—which is basically a mass of dead yeast. Some people like that smell and that taste—but for most people, it's not what they want from their sourdough.

A traditional starter can recover from either of the last two phases, because the starter is refreshed repeatedly and some microbes always survive. But with smart sourdough, the only remedy is to dump it and start over.

Luckily, it's not that hard to avoid these last phases. In fact, if you follow my instructions closely, you should never encounter them.

Stages of Smart Sourdough

Because there's no starter in smart sourdough, feeding cycles are spread over three basic stages of breadmaking. (Keep in mind that a new feeding cycle is triggered every time you add flour to your sourdough, no matter what else you're doing with it.)

Making the sponge. Some of the flour is mixed with all of the water to make a *sponge.* Setting the sourdough bacteria in such a wet environment helps them grow much more quickly than they would in normal dough. Still, the microbes take time to wake up, and the populations are starting from low levels, so this feeding cycle lasts the longest, taking close to half the recipe time to achieve good sourness.

Feeding the sponge. One or more times, the sponge is fed more flour to start a new cycle. This is done *without* discarding any of the sponge, which becomes more doughy with each feeding—less hydrated and more favoring production of acetic acid. At the kind of temperatures I recommend, a cycle of this type takes just a few hours.

Making the loaf. The remaining flour is added along with the yeast and any other ingredients, and the loaf is shaped and allowed to rise. Of course, this cycle has to end as soon as the loaf is properly risen, but we still want it to last long enough to generate more acetic acid. So, to extend the time, the yeast is added in only a tiny amount, making it take longer to multiply to normal strength.

With this simple approach, your sourdough reaches a good level of sourness by the time the loaf is ready for the oven—without starter and all within 24 hours!

The Right Setup

There are no warming devices designed just for heating sourdough. So, we have to figure out how to use the ones we have—and in many cases, how to *adapt* them for what we want.

That's what I've done—with some help from my clever wife—for a home proofer, slow cookers like the Instant Pot, and a sous vide cooker. If you own one of the devices featured in the sample setup sidebars following this chapter, you're in luck!—I've already done the hardest part for you. If you don't, this chapter and those sidebars will provide tips for setting up whatever you have. Plus, procedures I'll give at the end will guide you through testing it.

If getting the setup right seems a challenge, take heart! Once this is out of the way, the rest of making smart sourdough is dirt simple.

Temperatures—Optimums, Settings, Targets

Let's start by identifying the different *kinds* of temperatures we need to deal with. I've already discussed *optimum* temperatures for sourdough in the chapter "The Right Conditions." To recap, the ones I've based this book on are:

- For the sponge, 105°F (about 40°C)
- For the loaf, 100°F (38°C)

But as I said back then, these optimums are *not* what you set on your warming device. Partly that's because many such devices are designed only for temperatures much higher—temperatures that would quickly kill the sourdough microbes.

Setup Temperatures		
	OPTIMUM	**TARGET**
Sponge	105°F (about 40°C)	100°F (38°C)
Loaf	100°F (38°C)	95°F (35°C)

We need to trick these devices into heating at temperatures lower than their settings.

But the other complication is the extra heat produced by microbe activity in the sourdough itself. To adjust for this, your device setup needs to aim at temperatures *a few degrees lower* than the optimums.

I call these *target temperatures*. They're calculated simply by subtracting five degrees Fahrenheit (almost three degrees Celsius) from the optimums. That gives you:

- For the sponge, 100°F (38°C)
- For the loaf, 95°F (35°C)

While *optimum* temperatures are great for designing recipes and understanding what's going on with our microbes, *target* temperatures are the more practical figures we'll use to figure out device setups.

Heating Methods

To adapt warming devices for sourdough, we have to understand the different ways a device can convey heat. The fact is, warming devices often heat in more than one way at once!

Direct heating. This kind of heating—the main kind used by a slow cooker—is what you get when your sourdough or its container is in contact with hot surfaces of your device. For instance, if you mix and warm your sourdough directly in a Crock-Pot, or in the inner pot of an Instant Pot, you're using direct heating. If the sourdough is already in its own bowl when you place it in the device, that's still direct heating—but in a less efficient form, especially if the bowl is plastic or if its base isn't snug against the cooker floor.

In a Brød & Taylor home proofer, direct heating is what you get when you remove the rack and place your sourdough bowl on the metal heating plate. Brød & Taylor now calls this its Slow Cook Mode.

Direct heating is the quickest and most powerful kind of heat transfer. In fact, it's usually *too* powerful for sourdough. Unless a device has been designed for the more moderate temperatures that sourdough microbes prefer, direct heating will kill them. So, for instance, you can't put your sourdough directly in a Crock-Pot, even at the lowest setting, without cooking the microbes.

Even when a warming device *does* allow you to set a temperature low enough—as with the Instant Pot and its Yogurt setting (104°F, 40°C)—its heating element is likely too strong. This creates hot spots in your sourdough that can lead to runaway microbe growth. I'd hate to tell you how many times my sourdough experiments with that Yogurt setting have ended in stinking failures.

The moral, then, is to *avoid* warming sourdough with direct heating. But don't worry, that doesn't mean you can't use the device. It just means you can't use it *that way*. But it's not that hard to adapt such a device, as I'll discuss shortly.

Air heating. Conveying heat via heated air is the main way that ovens operate, whether it's a standard kitchen oven, or a countertop oven, or a convection oven. Because of the high temperatures that ovens need to reach, their heating elements are *way* too strong for sourdough. It's rare to find an oven that lets you set a temperature low enough—but even if you do, the oven's actual temperature will fluctuate far too widely.

Some sourdough bakers use a kitchen oven to quickly warm their sourdough, and then leave it there to ferment as the oven slowly cools. This can certainly work with some finagling—but for smart sourdough, you'll need a method that allows more control.

Another device that heats by air—often with more control and in a better temperature range—is a dehydrator. Some can be set down to 95°F (35°C) or even lower. But I haven't tried one myself, so you're on your own!

Steam heating. Steam is a great conveyor of heat—much better than air. You'll know about that if you've ever steamed vegetables or (less likely) used a steam oven.

With sourdough, a tiny amount of steam is often used to keep the loaf from crusting over as it rises. When doing that, though, you're less concerned about *warming* the sourdough with the steam than about keeping the steam from *overheating* it. In fact, if you're not careful, you can easily wind up killing off all your bacteria and yeast. I'll say more about that shortly.

Water heating. Better than air at conveying heat, and better again than steam, is water. Some of you will already know where this is heading: sous vide! With its flexible and precise temperature control, a sous vide cooker turns out to be a surprisingly effective way to warm sourdough. For the sponge, all you need to do is float your bowl in the water bath.

Here is the most interesting thing about water heating, and the biggest surprise from my sous vide experiments: Water is so efficient at conveying heat that it works in both directions!

The water in sous vide not only heats the sourdough quickly and precisely to the set temperature, it also *draws away* the extra heat generated by the sourdough itself. The sourdough temperature, then, never varies more than a degree or two from the setting on your cooker.

That makes sous vide the *only* method I've found that lets you set a chosen temperature and actually keep your sourdough very close to it.

Radiant heating. Finally we come to the workhorse of sourdough warming methods. Funny that most people have never heard of it!

All heated surfaces radiate heat in waves that travel unimpeded through air till they hit something solid. The hotter the radiating surface, the more heat it radiates. This way of heating is gentle and gradual, and you might not even notice its effect if a stronger form of heating is active at the same time. But when all on its own, it's just perfect for warming sourdough.

In the Brød & Taylor home proofer, you get radiant heating simply by placing your bowl or pan on the supplied rack—which sits about half an inch *above* the heating plate—instead of on the plate itself. Brød & Taylor now calls this its Proofer Mode.

Heating Methods by Strength

Radiant

Air

Steam

Water

Direct

The Brød & Taylor may well be the only good-sized kitchen appliance designed to warm primarily by radiant heating—which is what makes it uniquely suited to sourdough. But devices designed to heat by other methods can often be adapted to heat this way instead—as I'll discuss next.

Adapting Your Device

Chances are, if you own *any* warming device, you own an Instant Pot or other slow cooker. As I said, the direct heating used by these cookers is too strong for warming sourdough. But any of them can be converted to radiant heating just by lifting your bowl or pan away from the device's hot surface.

With the Instant Pot, for instance, you could place a small bowl with sourdough on a steamer rack in the inner pot—*without* adding water for steam. In fact, I experimented with this myself for quite some time. The drawback—as you can easily imagine—is that there's not much room in there. With most cookers, only a small bowl will fit, and forget about your loaf pan!

The solution? Surprisingly simple, once my wife and I worked it out. With any slow cooker, you can place a wire rack *on top* of it, and then set your bowl or pan on that. Then the bowl or pan can be any size you like. (You'll see what this looks like in the sidebar "Instant Pot Setup.")

By using a slow cooker for radiant heating instead of direct, you get around the problem of too-high temperature settings. Those settings are for the temperatures you get with direct heating. If you warm with radiant at the *same* settings, your sourdough temperatures will be *much* lower.

In fact, that's a little trick of the Brød & Taylor. Switching at the control panel from Slow Cook Mode to Proofer Mode doesn't actually reduce the heat generated by the element—

it only changes the temperature shown on the display! The real difference between modes comes from where you place your food—directly on the heating plate or sitting above it on the rack.

The wire rack technique can work with sous vide too. Just place the rack over your dishpan or other water container, turning the water itself into a radiant heat source. This is handy for heating a loaf pan, which you probably don't want to float on the water!

Adding Steam

For a rising loaf, heating the sourdough is not *all* we want from our warming device. We also want it to generate enough steam to keep the loaf from crusting over—something that's especially important with our long rising time.

First off, let's be clear what we mean by *steam*. Strictly speaking, steam is simply water in the form of vapor or gas. Though you get the most steam from boiling, you also get it from evaporation at *any* temperature. And it's *invisible* till bits of it start condensing back to water (at which point it's technically called *wet steam* instead).

The sticky part about generating enough steam for a loaf is we need *higher* heat to make the steam than we want for the sourdough! For devices with direct heating, here's the trick: We'll use that *direct* heating to make steam, while—at the same time and with the same device—we warm the loaf with more gentle *radiant* heating.

The Brød & Taylor actually has this arrangement built into the proofer, with its water tray that sits directly on the metal plate—*beneath* the rack that holds your sourdough. So, while you're warming your loaf with a target temperature of 95°F (35°C), the temperature of the water in the tray is much higher—around 115°F (46°C).

You can rig up much the same arrangement with any slow cooker by placing a small bowl of water on the cooker's floor while your sourdough sits above it. Just don't put the water *directly* into the cooker, or you'll get enough steam to cook your sourdough! (Here again, see the sidebar "Instant Pot Setup.")

For sous vide, of course, the problem almost solves itself. With the loaf sitting above heated water, you're already producing steam right below it!

Unless your loaf is in an enclosed space—as with a proofer—you'll need something to collect the rising steam. A cake cover over your loaf pan can work well for this. You can also devise your own cover—preferably transparent, so you can see inside.

Don't forget that steam will raise the temperature of your sourdough. So, you will likely need to lower the temperature setting of your warming device to compensate. Most important, you have to make sure there's not enough steam to overheat the sourdough and kill its microbes—which will start around 120°F (close to 50°C).

Though I've been able to find ways to generate steam with several warming devices, I won't say it's *always* possible. For instance, I don't know how I'd do it with a dehydrator—which is one reason I haven't tried one. But if you don't mind babysitting, you could forget steam entirely. In its place, you could cover the pan with cloth and use a mister on the loaf as needed.

Brød & Taylor Proofer Setup

Make & Model: Brød & Taylor Folding Proofer (first generation) or Folding Proofer & Slow Cooker (second generation). It's easy—and important—to tell the difference. The second generation includes a button on the control panel to toggle between Proofer Mode and Slow Cook Mode. The first generation has no separate modes, officially working only as a proofer.

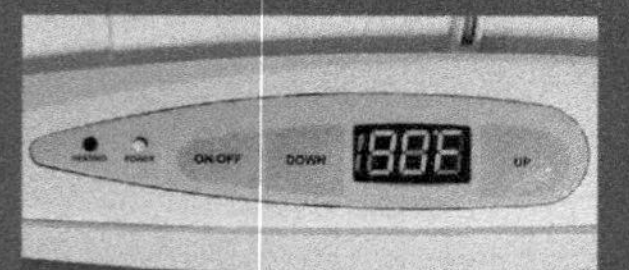

First generation

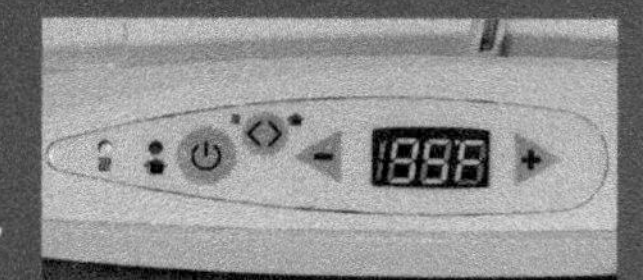

Second generation

Sponge Heating Method: Radiant

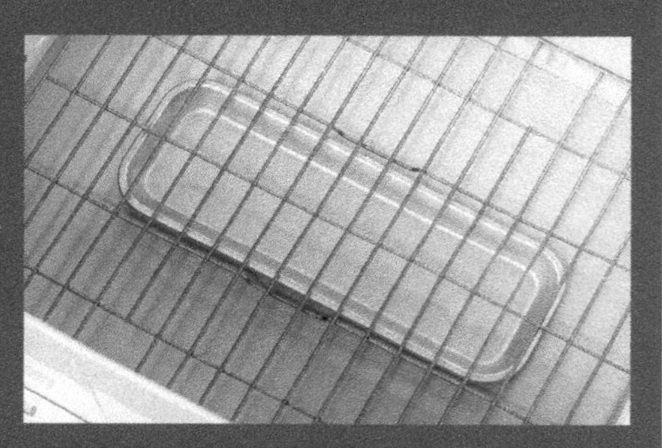

Sponge Setup: After raising the walls of the proofer, put the *empty* water tray—no water in it yet!—directly on the metal heating plate and centered on it. Put the wire rack in place above it, with the feet and central ridges pointing down and the tray nestled between the ridges. Place your mixing bowl with sponge on top of the rack, centered. Do not cover the bowl. Set the proofer lid in place.

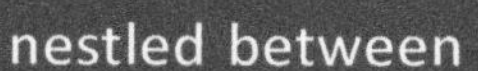

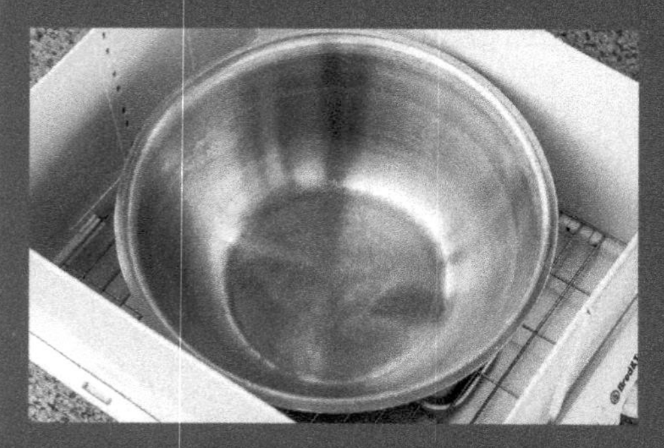

Sponge Setting: For the second-generation proofer, set the mode to Proofer. For the first *and* second generation, set the temperature to 100°F (38°C).

Loaf Heating Method: Radiant and steam

Loaf Setup: With your water tray still in place under the rack, pour water into it—about half a cup. Place your loaf pan on top of the rack, centered but at a *right angle* to the water tray—to avoid catching all the

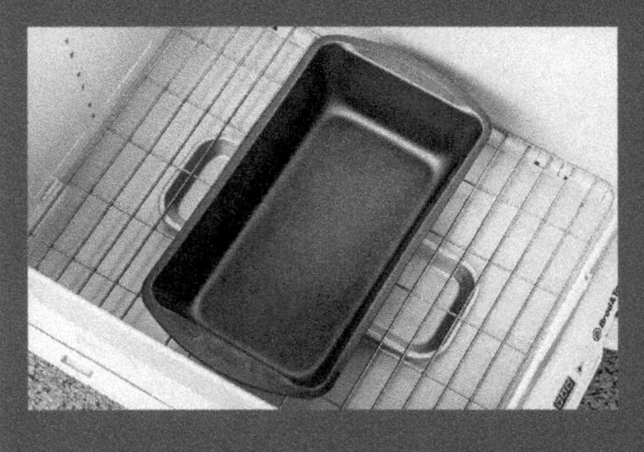

steam on the pan's underside. Do not cover the loaf pan. Set the proofer lid in place.

Loaf Setting: For the second-generation proofer—still in Proofer Mode—set the temperature to 95°F (35°C). For the first-generation proofer, set the temperature to 90°F (32°C)—a different setting for this model!

Notes

Temperatures were tested for a stainless steel mixing bowl and a steel loaf pan with a dark nonstick coating. (Brød & Taylor itself uses stainless steel containers to calibrate the proofer's temperature settings.)

Keep everything centered in the proofer, because that's where the heating plate is hottest.

Because the proofer warms mostly by radiant heating—unlike an oven, which heats mostly by air—you don't have to worry about the proofer enclosure not being airtight, or about losing heat when you lift the lid.

The wire rack's feet must point *up* when the proofer is folded for storing, but *down* when in use. In other words, when setting up *or* taking down, don't forget to turn the rack over!

The loaf temperature setting is different for the second generation proofer, because—*for any setting up to 95°F (35°C)*—it assumes you're using the water tray, and it *reduces* heat from the plate to make up for expected heat from steam. Sounds all right, as long as you really are using the water tray—which we happen to be, at that point. There's a catch, though: Since the proofer makes no such adjustment *above* that range, raising the setting just one degree beyond will produce a jump in sourdough temperature of *several* degrees. Mind the gap!

Instant Pot Setup

Make & Model: 6-quart Instant Pot Duo—but you'll find the same settings on *any* Instant Pot, and the basic setup should work for any Instant Pot or other slow cooker. (Setting some Instant Pot models to Keep Warm can be tricky, so see your user manual if needed.)

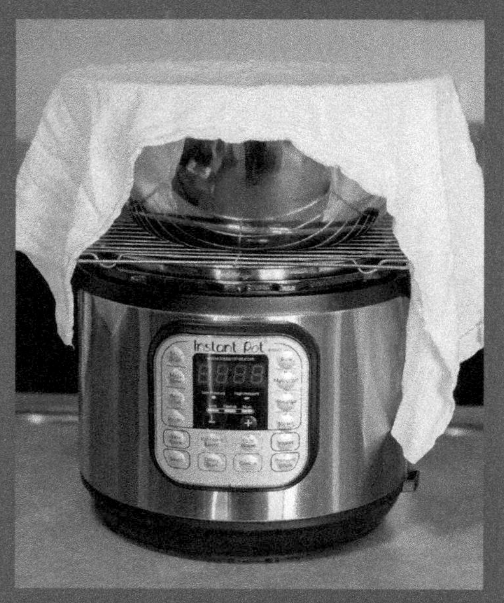

Sponge Heating Method: Radiant

Sponge Setup: With the Instant Pot lid removed, place a wire rack *on top* of the inner pot and set your mixing bowl with sponge on the rack. Cover the bowl with a dry flour sack towel or other cloth.

Sponge Setting: Slow Cook Normal

Loaf Heating Method: Radiant and steam

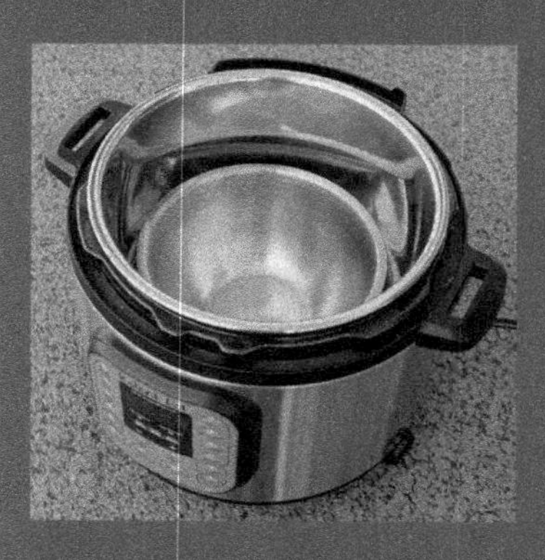

Loaf Setup: On the floor of the inner pot, place a small stainless steel bowl filled with one cup of *hot* water. Replace the rack on top of the pot and place your loaf pan on it. Cover the loaf pan with a cake cover or other cover that will catch steam.

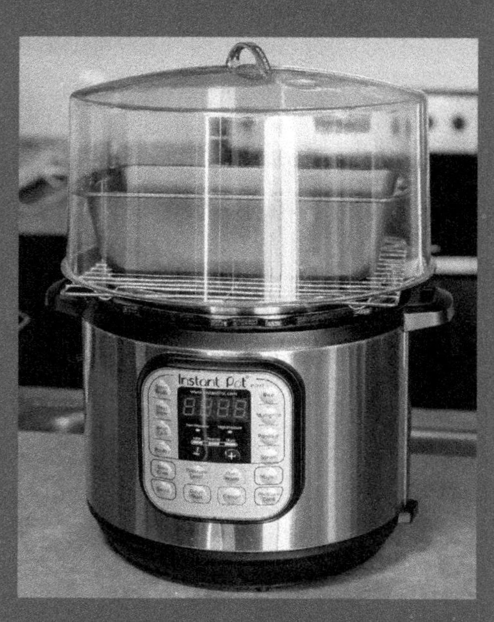

Loaf Setting: Keep Warm Normal

Notes

Temperatures were tested for a stainless steel mixing bowl and a steel loaf pan with a dark nonstick coating.

IMPORTANT! After a few minutes, the Instant Pot may display a "burn" error message on its control panel. But assuming nothing is actually burning, this is only to tell you there's not enough liquid in the pot to allow pressure cooking—which you're not using. In less than a minute, the message should disappear, and the Instant Pot should function normally.

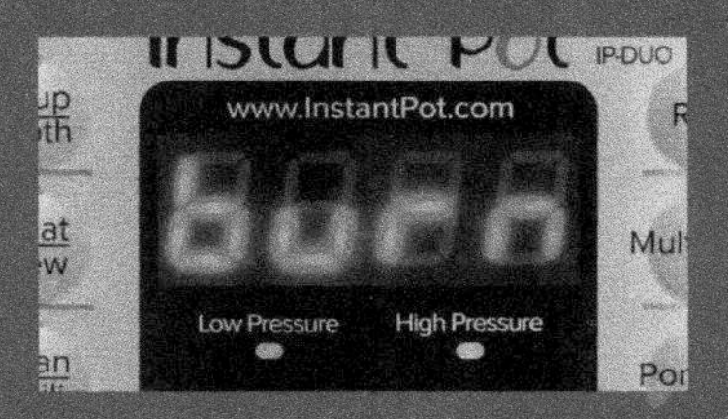

In Instant Pot manuals, the temperatures ascribed to my recommended settings are much higher than you want for your sourdough—but keep in mind that those are for *direct* heating. Since you're warming with *radiant* heating, the temperatures of your sourdough will be much lower.

The Instant Pot Duo is one model that has Less, Normal, and More levels for the Slow Cook and Keep Warm settings. Though the temperature differences between these levels are sizeable for direct heating, they're not that large for radiant. So, you can switch among them for small adjustments.

If your Instant Pot has only *one* level for a setting, it's the same as Normal.

To make steam for the loaf, do *not* put water directly in the cooker. That will cook your sourdough in no time!

Sous Vide Setup

Make & Model: Anova Nano Precision Cooker—but the setup and settings should work with any sous vide immersion circulator (aka portable stick model).

Sponge Heating Method: Water

Sponge Setup: Fill your dishpan or other container with water to within a few inches of the top. Attach your cooker in a corner of the container. Float your mixing bowl with sponge on the water. Cover the bowl with a dry flour sack towel or other cloth, draping the ends over the water container sides to keep the cloth from dipping into the sponge or the water. Now and then, check the water level to make sure it does not go below the cooker's minimum level.

Sponge Setting: 100°F (38°C)

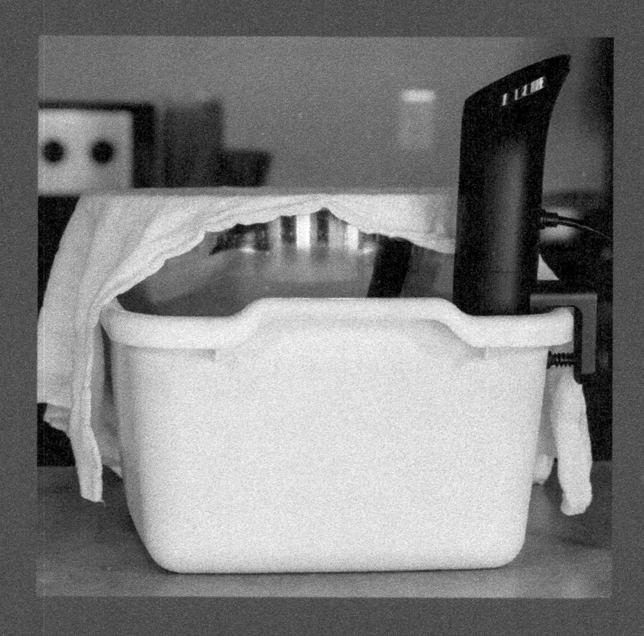

Loaf Heating Method: Radiant and steam

Loaf Setup: Place a wire rack over the water container and set your loaf pan on it. Cover the loaf pan with a cake cover or other cover that will catch steam.

Loaf Setting: 110°F (43°C)

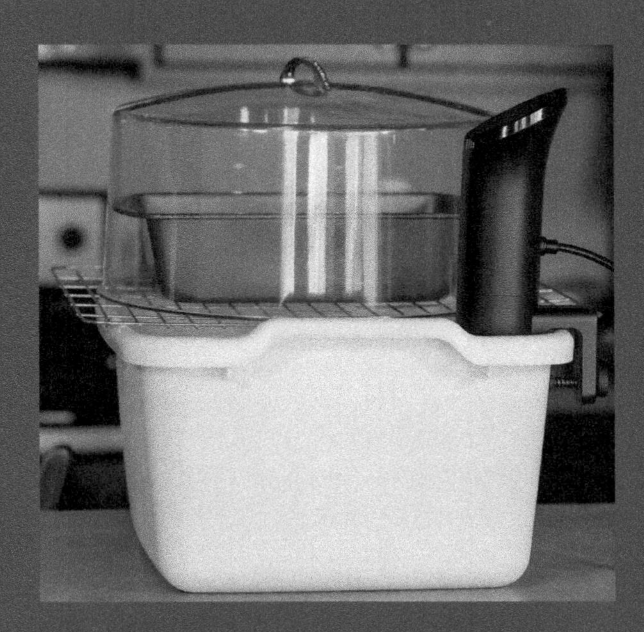

Notes

Temperatures were tested for a stainless steel mixing bowl and a steel loaf pan with a dark nonstick coating.

Note that the sous vide cooker and its heating by water will hold the sponge temperature *lower* than will other devices at equivalent settings. But it will also warm the sponge *more quickly*—so this should keep the recipe times the same.

Also note, because of the entirely different heating methods used for the loaf, the device setting for that is *higher* than for the sponge. (With most other devices, the setting for the loaf is lower.)

Testing Your Setup

Whether you're devising your own setup or using one of mine, you'll want to test it to make sure you're hitting the right temperatures. And because so many things affect temperature, you'll want to nail this *before* you start making bread.

Luckily, you should have to deal with this only once. Remember, though, you need to test *two* setups—one for the sponge and one for the loaf. The procedures that follow this sidebar will guide you through.

It's best to run your tests at least a day ahead, so you'll have time to let temperatures settle and to make your adjustments. Start with *exactly* the settings and setup you're thinking to use for your sourdough, right down to the covering (or lack of it) for your mixing bowl or loaf pan. The only difference is, you're going to heat water in place of sourdough.

Why water? Because here's where you get to work with those *target temperatures* I gave earlier—the ones that remove the factor of heat added by the sourdough itself. Basically, you can think of these targets as the temperatures that *water* should reach with the right settings and setup on your warming device.

Though your real sourdough will increase in volume with each feeding, you can approximate for testing with a constant amount of water throughout. I use three cups.

If you can't quite get your water to a target temperature even after adjustment, you may have to settle for "good enough." If the temperature is a little low, chances are the chief impact will be only that you'll need longer fermenting times.

Landing too high, though, can be more of a problem. If your test water reaches 110°F (43°C), added heat from microbe activity can carry temperatures into the range where microbes die. And for the loaf, a test temperature over 105°F (about 40°C) will later mean weakened yeast and a slower rise. So, if you have a choice between too low or too high, too low is the safer choice.

Sponge Setup Test

Target temperature: 100°F (38°C)

1. Start with 3 cups of water in your mixing bowl at close to room temperature. Measure the water temperature in the center of the bowl with your folding thermometer and record the reading.
2. Begin heating the bowl of water with your warming device, using the setup and setting you hope will bring that water to this test's target temperature.
3. Measure the temperature again about every half hour and record the readings. Continue till the temperature has changed no more than one degree in half an hour.
4. If the temperature settles within a degree or two of your target, take note of the setup and setting and use it for your sponge when making sourdough. If it doesn't reach the target—or if it overshoots—adjust as needed and test again. (The water does not have to start over at room temperature.)
5. If your testing goes into a second day, top off the water to replace any lost to evaporation.

Tips: With most devices, the temperature should rise faster at first, then gradually slow down before leveling off. All together, this might take a couple of hours or so.

Adjusting for a temperature too low or too high might be as simple as changing your device's temperature setting by the difference in degrees. But if you're adapting a direct heat device for radiant heating, you'll probably need to change the setting by *more* than that. (Try doubling the difference.) Meanwhile, some devices, like the Instant Pot, don't even *allow* continuous temperature adjustment. A device like that might not have *any* setting that's exactly right.

In that case, you may have to change part of your setup. With radiant heating, for example, a glass mixing bowl will absorb more heat, while shiny stainless steel will absorb less. Also, you can increase or reduce the effect of radiant heating by moving the bowl closer to or farther from the heated surface. (See the chapter "The Right Setup" for more on adjustments.)

Loaf Setup Test

Target temperature: 95°F (35°C)

1. Transfer your test water from your mixing bowl to your loaf pan, or start fresh with 3 cups of water in the pan. (The water does not have to start at room temperature.) Measure the water temperature in the center of the pan with your folding thermometer and record the reading. If you plan to generate steam to prevent crusting of the loaf, put water for that in your chosen container.
2. Begin heating the loaf pan of water with your warming device, using the setup and setting you hope will bring that water to this test's target temperature and generate the needed steam.
3. Measure the temperature again about every half hour and record the readings. Continue till the temperature has changed no more than one degree in half an hour.
4. If the temperature settles within a degree or two of your target—and if the amount of steam generated seems about right—take note of the setup and setting and use it for your loaf when making sourdough. If it doesn't reach the target—or if it overshoots—or if there seems to be too much or too little steam—adjust as needed and test again.
5. If your testing goes into a second day, top off the water to replace any lost to evaporation.

Tips: Your target temperature for the loaf is *lower* than for the sponge—so, depending on how you start, you may be watching your water temperature fall instead of rise. Either way, the aim is to wait till it settles.

You can adjust temperature for your loaf setup basically the same ways you did for your sponge setup. Remember, though, that the steam too is heating your test water. (See the chapter "The Right Setup" for more on adjustments.)

Final adjustment of your steam generation may have to wait till you can see how well it's preventing crusting of your loaf. In general, though, if you're using a transparent cover to collect the steam, you want to see a light misting on that cover without your view being completely blocked.

The best way to adjust the steam amount would be to switch your water container. With direct heating, for example, you'll get more steam from a container that's wider and that fits more snugly against the heated surface. Changing the *amount* of water in the container may change how quickly the steam starts appearing.

Of course, with a change in the amount of steam, you'll have to check also for a change of temperature in your test water.

Making Smart Sourdough

We're finally ready to begin baking! To start you off, here is my basic recipe—a 50% whole wheat sandwich loaf.

The recipe gives you a single large loaf of about 2¼ pounds (about 1 kilogram). If you're baking just for yourself and have good self-control, that's enough for a sandwich a day for a week, plus maybe a slice to enjoy while the loaf is still warm from the oven. If you're baking for a family, or you have low willpower . . . Well, it probably won't last long!

Total time for the recipe, start to finish, is about 20 hours, plus a few hours for cooling. Actual work time should be an hour or less, including cleanup. The recipe is timed roughly so you can start your sourdough in the evening, let it sit overnight, continue the next morning and afternoon, and have warm bread for supper—but figure exact timing based on when you're awake and available. See the Sample Schedules chart for suggestions.

This basic recipe is what I call a *four-cycle sourdough*, because it includes four feeding cycles—the initial making of the sponge, the final adding of flour for the loaf, and two feedings in between. The taste of a sourdough like this could turn out as anything from "sweet" to mildly sour—though you can adjust the sourness by several methods, as I'll describe in the chapter "Customizing Your Sourdough."

As is common in bread recipes, the ingredients here and in later recipes are listed with the flour first—in this case, beginning with the whole grain—with the remaining ingredients shown in order of addition.

Sample Schedules

	"EARLY RISER"	"MIDDLE WAY"	"NIGHT OWL"
Prepare ingredients	7:00 p.m.	8:00 p.m.	10:00 p.m.
Make sponge	9:00 p.m.	10:00 p.m.	12:00 a.m.
Feed sponge (1)	6:00 a.m.	7:00 a.m.	9:00 a.m.
Feed sponge (2)	9:00 a.m.	10:00 a.m.	12:00 p.m.
Make loaf	12:00 p.m.	1:00 p.m.	3:00 p.m.
Bake	3:00 p.m.	4:00 p.m.	6:00 p.m.

If the amount of water seems high to you—it is! You *need* to add too much, because a lot of it will evaporate at these temperatures—up to half a cup.

Please don't agonize over getting the measured amounts exact. There are so many variables in sourdough—who knows?—a little variance might actually improve your result!

On the other hand—at least the first time—try to resist any urge to purposely change the recipe or combine my method with others. That way, if you do make changes later, you'll know if they're the cause of any problems.

Whole wheat flour used in testing this recipe—and later ones—included King Arthur White Whole Wheat Flour, King Arthur Whole Wheat Flour, and homeground white wheat. Unbleached bread flour included King Arthur Unbleached Bread Flour and King Arthur Organic Unbleached Bread Flour.

About Recipe Sketches

After mastering the method in my basic recipe, you'll use basically the same method for all other sourdough recipes in this book! To avoid page after page of repetition, I've come up with a shorthand recipe form I call a *recipe sketch*. It gives you only the changeable details of the recipe, so you can plug them back into the basic method.

The recipe sketch shown here is both an overview and a summary of the full recipe that follows it. For greater convenience, make a copy of the sketch and jot in the time you should start each cycle.

Smart Sourdough

50% WHOLE WHEAT—LARGE LOAF—4 CYCLES

12 ounces whole wheat flour, 12 ounces unbleached bread flour, extra flour for kneading, 2½ cups water, 2 teaspoons salt, ⅛ teaspoon yeast

Sponge: 12 ounces whole wheat flour, 2½ cups water, 2 teaspoons salt
Warm with a target of 100°F (38°C) for 9 hours.

1st Feeding: 4 ounces unbleached bread flour
Warm with a target of 100°F (38°C) for 3 hours.

2nd Feeding: 4 ounces unbleached bread flour
Warm with a target of 100°F (38°C) for 3 hours.

Loaf: 4 ounces unbleached bread flour, extra flour for kneading, ⅛ teaspoon yeast
Warm and steam with a target of 95°F (35°C) for about 3 hours.

Bake at 375°F (190°C) for 45 minutes from a cold oven.

This is a "recipe sketch" of the full recipe that follows.

Smart Sourdough

12 ounces whole wheat flour
12 ounces unbleached bread flour, divided
Extra flour for kneading
2½ cups water
2 teaspoons salt
⅛ teaspoon yeast, active dry or instant

Tips: See the chapter "The Right Ingredients" for details on selection.

In the United Kingdom, bread flour is called *strong flour*.

If you're not concerned with maximizing the rise, all-purpose flour can be substituted for bread flour—as long as it's not a low-protein brand, as may be found in the southern United States.

The "extra flour for kneading" can be your choice—whole wheat, unbleached bread flour, or something different.

If you have good access to high extraction flour—as you might in the United Kingdom or mainland Europe—you should be able to substitute it for *all* the flour.

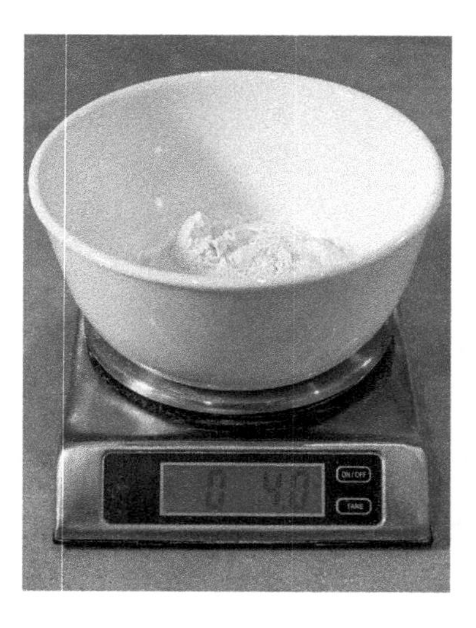

The ounce measurements for flour are by weight—not volume!—and require a scale accurate to a tenth of an ounce. (See the earlier sidebar "Why Weigh Your Flour?" to explain why no cup measurements are given.) If you're already weighing flour, you might be used to grams instead of ounces—but your scale should switch easily from one to the other, and tenths of an ounce are more than precise enough for sourdough.

The amount of water given is the *most* you'll likely need. The *exact* amount needed can vary—depending on evaporation and your flour's moisture content—but the "extra flour for kneading" makes up the difference. Still, if you find you need more than a few extra ounces for kneading, you can try reducing the water the next time.

If your yeast is old and weak, the rise may take longer than expected. A bit longer rise will not hurt the bread, but you can avoid it the next time by increasing the yeast amount. (Doubling the yeast cuts rising time about three-quarters of an hour.)

Advance Setup

Suggested time: Day before first time, and before other times as needed

1. Test your warming device, following the directions at the end of the chapter "The Right Setup."
2. Fill a pitcher or other large container with water and set it out to reach room temperature and to let chlorine evaporate.
3. Sanitize your mixing bowl and kitchen spoon in your dishwasher, with your hottest tap water, or with 70% isopropyl alcohol.

Tips: Details on warming devices and setting them up can be found in the chapters "The Right Equipment" and "The Right Setup."

Top off your pitcher later as needed to keep chlorine-free, room-temperature water always handy.

Sanitizing the bowl and spoon is done only to ensure more predictable results by starting with a nearly clean microbial slate. It is *not* normally needed for safety. You can later do this step as part of your cleanup. (Or purposely avoid it, as proposed later in the sidebar "Smart Cleanup.")

Preparing the Ingredients

Suggested time: Early evening

1. Measure out the 2½ cups of water into a large measuring cup or jar. Add the 2 teaspoons of salt to the water, then stir or swish briefly to help the salt dissolve.

2. For making the sponge, weigh out the 12 ounces of whole wheat flour into your mixing bowl. If needed, cover the bowl.

3. For feeding the sponge and making the loaf, weigh out the 12 ounces of unbleached bread flour into three smaller bowls, with 4 ounces in each bowl. If needed, cover the bowls.

4. Extra flour for kneading—though not weighed—should be left out, rather than refrigerated, to be at room temperature when needed.

5. If needed, wait an hour or two for the flour in your mixing bowl to approach room temperature before you proceed. To cut the time, you can warm it in your microwave or cool it in your refrigerator, but be careful not to overshoot. (And do not place a metal bowl in the microwave.)

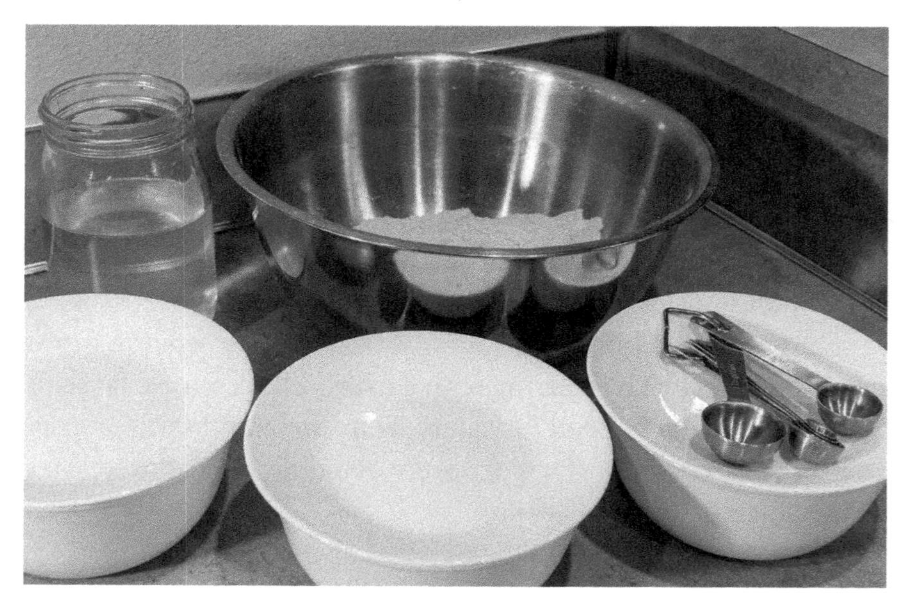

Tips: If you're grinding your own whole wheat flour, you can do that as a first step. Weigh the wheat berries before grinding to save you weighing the flour later.

See the sidebar "Starting with Salt" for why it's added early.

To disregard the weight of a bowl and start weighing the flour from zero, place the bowl on the scale *before* turning it on, or press Tare to reset.

It's a good idea to place your measuring spoons in or on the smaller bowl of flour you mean to use last. This will remind you to add yeast before making the loaf—something easy to forget!

Making the Sponge

Suggested time: Late evening

1. Stir or swish the salt water again, then pour it into the flour in the mixing bowl. Mix thoroughly with a kitchen spoon. DO NOT ADD THE YEAST NOW.
2. With your warming device set up for a sponge, place your mixing bowl in or on it and begin heating the sponge to the target temperature of 100°F (38°C). Cover your bowl *only* if it's exposed to the open air, and then only with cloth.
3. Leave the sponge to ferment for 9 hours. During this time, avoid stirring the sponge or disturbing its surface.

Tips: The later chapter "Testing Your Sourdough" will tell you how to judge your sponge's progress. At the end of nine hours, it should give signs of souring—but if not, don't worry too much. The sponge can still "catch up" in later cycles.

Because of the high proportion of water to flour, timing for this cycle is more critical than for the others, as microbe activity is more intense. An extra hour here could ruin your sponge.

Starting with Salt

The conventional wisdom for sourdough is that salt should be added as late as possible, and certainly never when making the sponge, because it inhibits growth of the sourdough microbes. But as I've said, it inhibits those microbes' competitors even more, paving the way for your favored ones. So, when aiming at quick and reliable souring, it's best to add salt *at the very beginning*.

This is not really different from natural pickling, where vegetables are submerged in brine—salty water—to create a favorable environment for lactic acid bacteria—the same kind of bacteria that make sourdough sour.

There's another reason to add salt sooner. One of the purposes of making a sponge is to help develop gluten strands for better rising. Salt helps that development.

What's more, if you instead wait and mix salt into a sponge *after* those strands have developed, the edges of the salt crystals cut the strands—so you lose much of what you gained. If you've ever mixed salt into a day-old sponge, you've probably watched it grow runnier as you stirred. Better, then, to add the salt early, so it's dissolved *before* the strands develop.

We do, though, want to minimize the effect of the salt on the sourdough bacteria. After all, direct contact with salt can kill them. The solution, then, is to dissolve the salt before it goes into the sponge! And that's what I do in my recipe, mixing the salt with the water beforehand.

Truthfully, when and how you add your salt is not likely to make or break your sourdough. Still—especially in a 24-hour method—it just makes sense to give your sourdough bacteria the best conditions you can.

Feeding the Sponge

Suggested time: Early and late morning

1. Remove the sponge from your warming device and add the 4 ounces of flour from one of your smaller bowls. Thoroughly stir in the flour with your kitchen spoon.
2. Return the sponge to your warming device and leave it to ferment for another 3 hours. During this time, avoid stirring the sponge or disturbing its surface.
3. Repeat for the second feeding.

Tips: For these feedings, there's no need to add the flour gradually. Just dump it in and stir.

To avoid waste after stirring, you can scrape the sourdough off your kitchen spoon with a dinner spoon, returning the scrapings to the sponge.

Making the Loaf

Suggested time: Early afternoon

1. *Lightly* oil or grease your loaf pan, or line it with parchment paper.
2. Remove the sponge from your warming device. Without giving it much time to cool, stir it just enough to break up the top crust and mix in the pieces. Then sprinkle the ⅛ teaspoon of yeast over the sponge and stir it in thoroughly with your kitchen spoon.
3. Gradually add flour from the 4 ounces in the last of your smaller bowls, stirring it in with your kitchen spoon, till the dough stops sticking to the mixing bowl.

4. Knead the dough by hand for up to several minutes while adding any remaining flour from the smaller bowl plus any extra needed. You can stop when the dough is fairly smooth and slightly springy.

5. Place the dough with seam down in your loaf pan. Spread the dough to the ends of the pan by pressing down in the center with the backs of your hands.

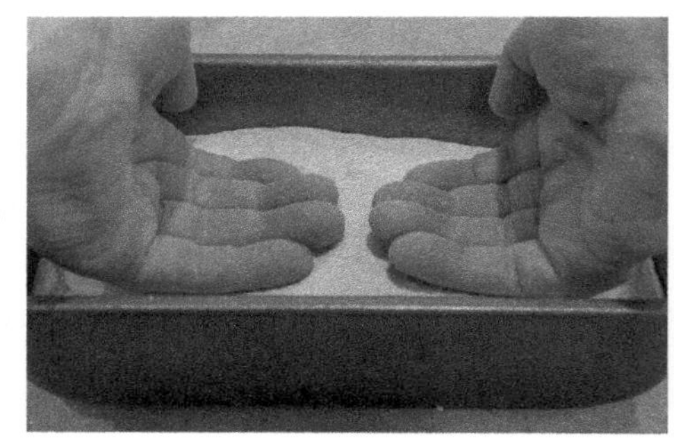

6. With your warming device set up for a loaf, place your loaf pan in or on it and begin heating the loaf to the target temperature of 95°F (35°C). For setups with steaming, remember to supply the needed water, and do *not* lay anything on the loaf pan to cover it. For setups *without* steaming, cover the pan with cloth.

7. Leave the loaf to ferment and rise for 3 hours or until the height doubles. For setups *without* steaming, occasionally use a mister with water to minimize crusting.

Tips: For reasons to knead by hand, a trick to minimize mess, and other tips, see the sidebar "The Joy of Kneading."

If you forgot and refrigerated your extra flour for kneading, you can bring it closer to room temperature in the microwave.

Your loaf should initially fill the pan about halfway. Almost all the rise will occur in the last hour. The loaf is ready to bake when its rising begins to slow—*before* the loaf reaches maximum height. Over-rising will later cause collapse in the oven.

With conventional breads, a second rise is favored to buy time for gluten development. Because of this recipe's long fermenting and rising times, you won't need that here.

The Joy of Kneading

Mix and knead the dough manually? Do I really tell you to do that? How primitive! Why not use a stand mixer or food processor?

Assuming you're not limited physically, here's why not:

1. Sourdough bacteria are mostly anaerobic, meaning they don't like oxygen. Machines mix in too much oxygen, slowing down bacteria growth.
2. With a machine, it's easy to overheat your dough or overwork your gluten. By hand, that's almost impossible.
3. After hand kneading, you can shape the loaf immediately instead of letting the dough rest.
4. With the sponge method and such long sitting times, no more than a few minutes of kneading are required.
5. For many of us, hand kneading is the most enjoyable part of breadmaking!

Then again, some of you may be asking yourself, why knead at all? Because:

1. Recipes that don't require kneading are for bread with huge holes—not the best if you hope to spread anything on your bread or make sandwiches.
2. See #4 and #5 under reasons not to use a machine.

Some cooking writers expound on the benefits of treating dough gently, so as not to injure the gluten or lose the dough's precious carbon dioxide and other gases. Well, during baking, those gases are forced out by heat and steam anyway, and as for the gluten, the best way to develop it is to press it against itself forcefully—in other words, to knead the dough. It's bread, not a baby!

I do understand, though, wanting to avoid the *mess* of kneading. While kneading is my favorite part of breadmaking, cleanup is my *least* favorite. So, I knead my dough right in the same big bowl

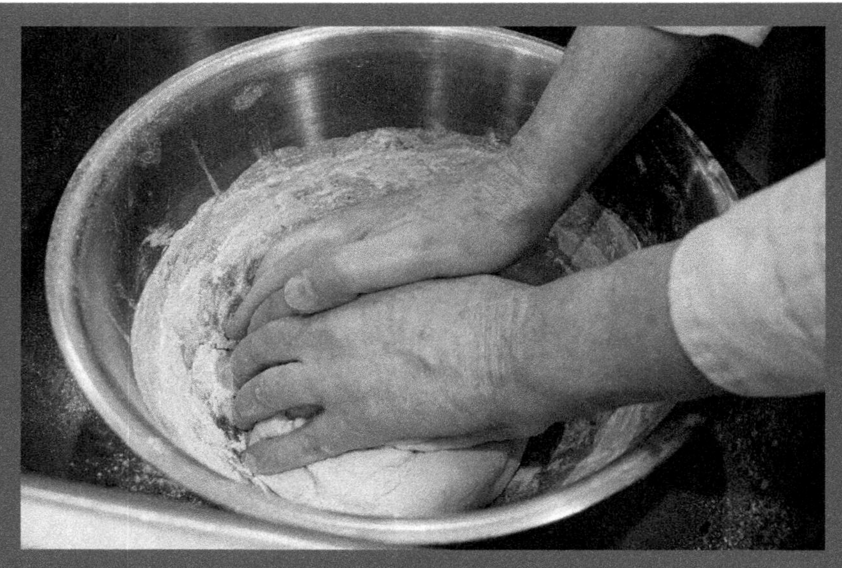

in which I mix it, with the bowl placed in the sink. The flour stays mostly in the bowl, and almost none escapes the sink, so it's easy to clean up.

There are many perfectly fine ways to knead dough, and if you need a demonstration, you'll find no shortage of videos online. What works well for me is to fold the dough over towards myself, press down on it with one hand over the other, rotate the dough a quarter turn, and repeat. It's practically all one motion, easier to do than to describe!

Throw loose flour under the dough as needed to keep it from sticking, and keep your hands floured as well. Oh, and remove your hand jewelry to keep it clean and to stop it from bruising your fingers. When kneading in the bowl, the main trick is to keep your fingers curled so the tips don't get jammed against the side.

I used to knead till the dough was fighting back, and I would measure its readiness partly by my own grunting. But with a long rise and pan baking, that's really not needed—and besides, if you keep adding flour, you'll wind up with a drier, heavier loaf. All you really need is to get the dough fairly smooth and a little springy. A couple of minutes should do it. Even a strenuous knead, though, shouldn't take more than five minutes.

Baking the Loaf

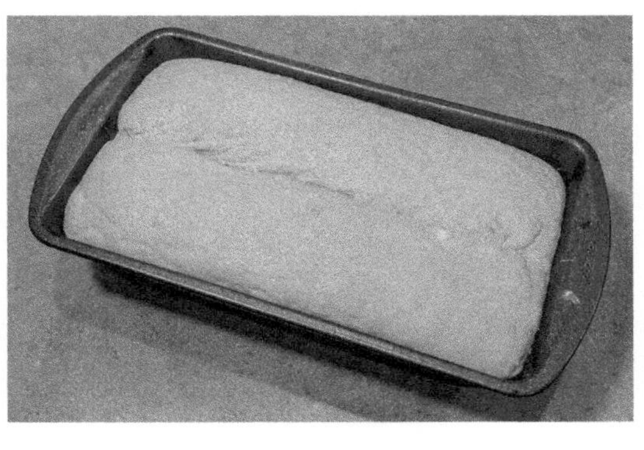

Suggested time: Late afternoon

1. Remove the loaf from your warming device. With the tip of a wet blade, make a slash down the length of the loaf to let it expand during baking.
2. *Starting from a cold oven,* bake the loaf in its pan on a middle shelf at 375°F (190°C) for 45 minutes.
3. Remove the loaf from the oven and check the temperature at its center to make sure it's at least 200°F (93°C). If it's too low, return the loaf to the oven for a few minutes and check again.
4. When the loaf has reached the desired temperature or above, remove it from the pan and cool it on a rack for several hours.

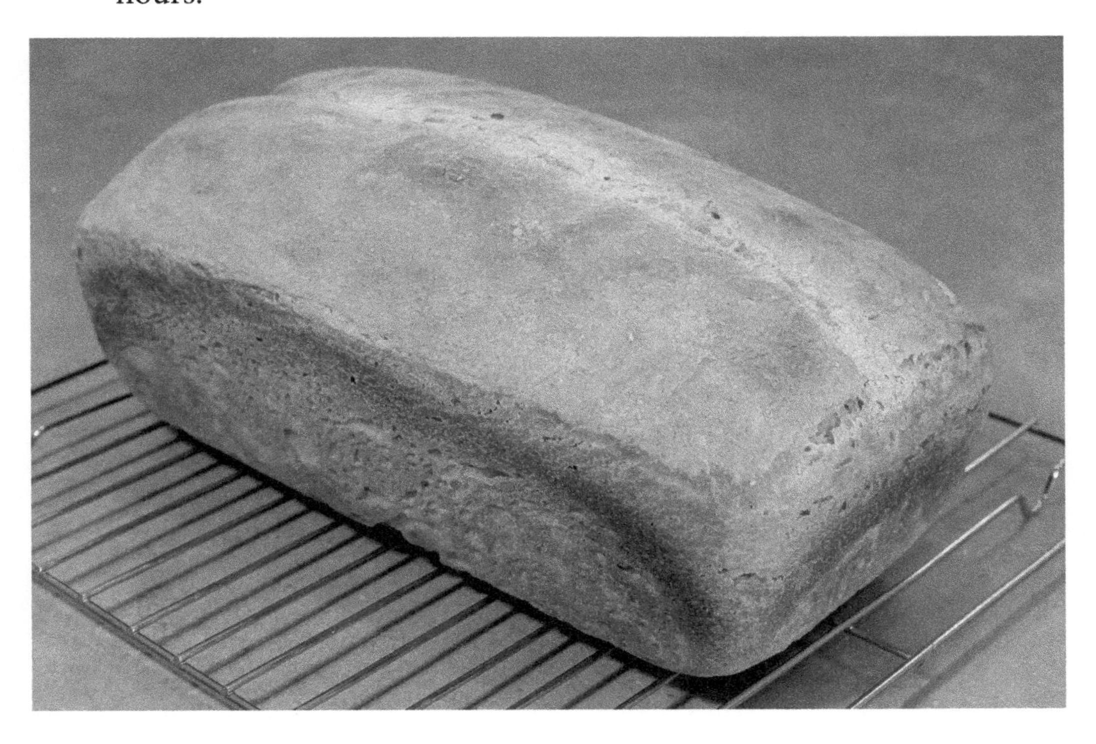

Tips: Starting from a cold oven is the simplest way to get maximum "oven spring" before the crust forms. To give a rough idea, this extra rise in a conventional electric oven will typically occur in the first quarter hour—about the same time the oven takes to reach its set temperature. For more on oven spring and other changes in a loaf as it bakes, see the sidebar "Oven Enigmas."

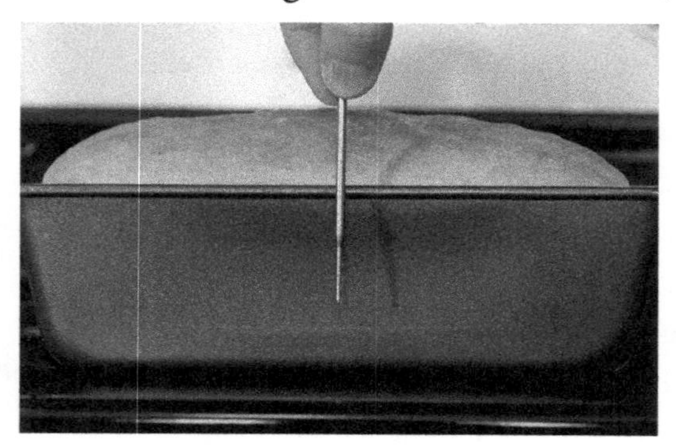

To insert the thermometer to the proper depth, first hold it *in front* of the loaf pan. With your eye on the same level, sight the point where the stem should stop going into the loaf and grab the stem there. Then insert the stem into the loaf, stopping just before your fingers hit the top.

It's easy to forget to turn off the oven after your final temperature check. To remind yourself, you can turn on the oven light when you turn on the oven, then leave the light on till you turn the oven off.

If the loaf does not fall out of your upside-down pan, try tapping one end against a hard surface. For more stubborn cases, you may need to slide a dinner knife or other flat implement between the loaf sides and the pan, doing your best not to mar the pan surface.

As a special treat, you can cut slices to eat after just one hour. (The bread is not "still cooking," as some bakers like to say, though the gluten will stiffen more as the bread cools.) If you do this, stand the loaf on its open end on a solid surface to trap moisture while the loaf is still cooling.

Oven Enigmas

Now for some fun. Here's a pop quiz you can take while you wait for your loaf to bake!

As your loaf starts to heat up in the oven, it rises higher, in what's commonly called *oven spring*. Any idea why this occurs?

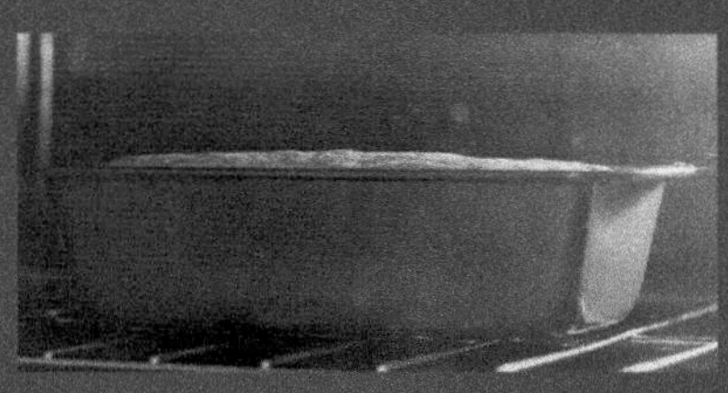

Oven spring, before . . .

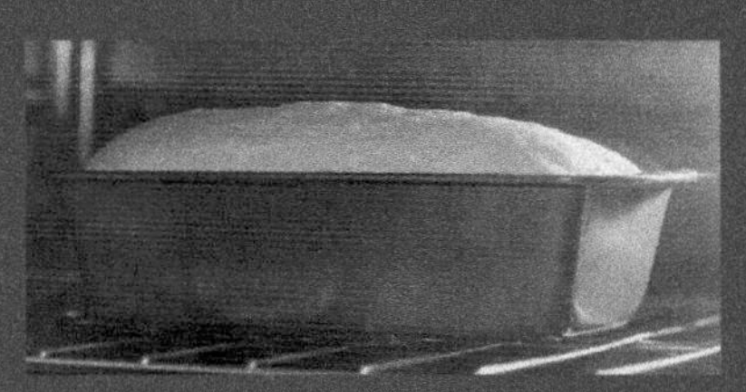

. . . and after

If you answered that oven heat gives the yeast a final spurt—Sorry! Wrong answer! Though that's the common belief, baker's yeast actually produces *less* gas for the rise as the temperature goes above 95°F (35°C), and the yeast's *growth* slows down even earlier.

No, what gives the loaf most of its final rise is *steam*. As the temperature rises, water in the loaf becomes steam, which fills the gas pockets created in the gluten by the yeast and expands them. In other words, the final rise is produced by the same force that makes popcorn pop. You might say that the pre-bake rise from the yeast is really just preparing for this final event.

That question leads to another: What's the best way to *help* oven spring?

I'm sure many of you are thinking "steam"—but this time, steam to fill the oven, which you can generate in a variety of ways. Many expert bakers do tell us that steam is needed to keep the crust from setting before the final rise is complete. But what those experts do *not* mention is that their ovens are on *all day.*

Since their ovens are super hot when they slide in the bread, these bakers do need steam to keep the crust soft at first. But most of us don't. All we need is to start from a cold oven. This gives the bread a good quarter hour or so to rise before the crust starts to form. It's really that simple, at least for a pan bread.

That's not the only advantage to starting from a cold oven. Another is that your loaf won't over-rise on your kitchen counter as it waits for the oven to preheat. Also, you'll save the cost of heating an oven with nothing yet in it.

Here's another question: How long does bread need to stay at its "done" temperature in order to bake properly?

Answer: It doesn't! The changes that transform dough into bread take place as the dough *reaches* certain temperatures. Once the loaf reaches its "done" temperature—around 200°F (around 93°C) in the center—all the changes you want are already finished! So, there's no need to keep it there.

Okay, one last question: If it takes five minutes in the oven for the temperature of your bread to rise from 175°F to 200°F, how long does it take for it to rise from 200°F to 225°F?

I have to admit, I don't know the exact answer myself—but it's a trick question anyway. Once the bread gets above 200°F (93°C), it's losing a lot of moisture as steam, and that carries away excess heat. And when it gets around 210°F (around 99°C)—just below water's boiling point—the temperature stops rising! It won't start again till the loaf dries out.

What's the lesson in this? If your baking time isn't exact, there's less risk in baking a few minutes too long than a few minutes too little.

Storing the Loaf

Suggested time: Evening

1. After the entire loaf has reached room temperature, bag it in plastic.
2. Leave it at room temperature for at least the first week. Do not cut slices before you need them.

Tips: *Do not bag the loaf till it is completely cool, or the crust will soften and the bread will mold.* Your plastic bag should be brand new or else washed in water hot enough to kill mold spores. If you won't be around to bag the loaf within a few hours after it has cooled, wrap it before that in cloth to slow down moisture loss till you can get to it.

Refrigerating or freezing the bread will dry it out, so avoid those if you can. The bread's high acidity should let it last at least a week at room temperature without spoiling, and possibly much longer. If spots of mold do appear, just slice them off and refrigerate after that. As the loaf loses freshness, you can partly refresh individual slices by toasting them, or an entire loaf by "rebaking."

Bread is best cut with a serrated knife. If you're not used to slicing bread by hand, your slices will become more even with practice.

Smart Cleanup

In case you've never cleaned utensils you've used to mix a sponge or dough, here's a warning: Don't put them straight into the dishwasher, and don't try cleaning them with a brush or scrubber! The gluten can really gum things up.

Instead, fill the mixing bowl with warm water—not hot, because you don't want to cook the dough. Put in the kitchen spoon too and let them both soak at least an hour. Then scrape off the dough by hand—and when I say "by hand," I mean literally with the fingers of your bare hand! Or you can use a bowl scraper, if you have one handy.

Your dishwasher or a brush or scrubber can handle the final residue. Your dishwasher will also sanitize the utensils—or you can do that just by filling the bowl with the hottest water from your tap. Or if you want to get extreme, you can wipe them with a clean cloth or paper towel doused with 70% isopropyl alcohol.

While working on this book, I scrupulously sanitized my mixing bowl and kitchen spoon between bakings. That's because I wanted to make sure that microbes from a previous test would not skew results from the next. And I suggest you do the same, at least at first, while getting the hang of smart sourdough.

This is a good place to admit, though, that I used to do something very different—and that I may go back to it. Instead of sanitizing my stainless steel mixing bowl, or even cleaning it down to bare metal, I kept hot water away from it and *purposely* left some residue. In other words, I kept it coated with a thin culture of sourdough microbes.

Of course, these microbes would dry out, but some apparently survived in that state, as many microbes do. And these survivors, which far outnumbered the microbes in fresh flour, were ready to jump to the task of souring my next sponge.

I called this my "starter bowl." I had a "starter spoon" too—not the soulless one made of easy-to-clean nylon I used for this book, but a good old-fashioned wooden spoon, riddled with microscopic pores where sourdough microbes could secretly stow away. As with the bowl, I kept it away from hot water and cleaned it only lightly by hand.

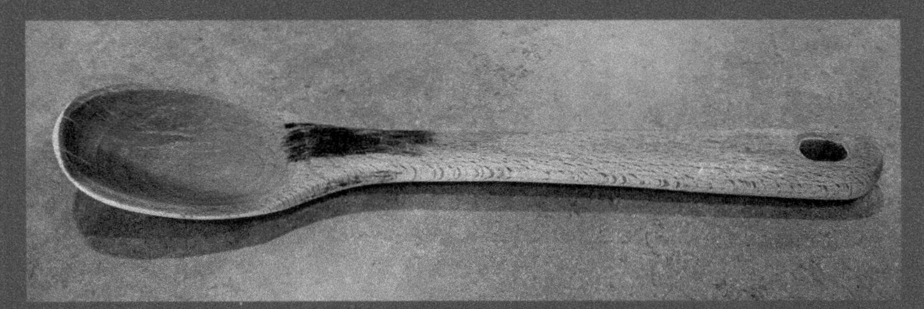

The advantage to using such "starters"? They can cut the length of the first feeding cycle by *hours*. Though I was mixing the sponge in the evening, I didn't put it in my proofer till the next morning, yet the sponge turned sour before lunch. Meanwhile, these "starters" required zero maintenance—not even refrigeration! All I had to do was make sure I used that bowl and that spoon for nothing but sourdough.

Obviously, you have to make sourdough at least once before you can even try this trick. That's one reason it has no part in my basic recipe, and why I stopped using it myself while testing for this book. But once you master the basic method, it's something you might like to try.

Testing Your Sourdough

We've already looked at how to test your warming device. Now here are some other tests you can use to troubleshoot your sourdough, or try new ideas, or just see what's going on.

Basic Tests

These are the tests I'm most likely to use when trying a change in recipe or when just baking for myself. They give me a good sense of how the sourdough is progressing.

Smell. If you know the bland smell of flour and water when they're first mixed, you can easily tell the difference after the sponge has come alive with fermentation—a smell that may not be quite sour but is at least enticingly tangy.

The sponge might start giving off this smell about an hour before the time for its first feeding. Generally, I catch the smell by sniffing at the edges of my folding proofer. Sometimes, though, I get a faint whiff from halfway across the room! Other times, I can't smell much at all even close to the bowl, but then I get a hit when stirring the sponge.

This semi-sour smell means your sourdough is well on its way. But there's another smell you can encounter that means it has gone way too far. If your sponge smells putrid, it probably means it has run out of food and you're stuck with a soup of dead and decomposing microbes.

If you've followed my instructions and recipe carefully, you will likely never get such a smell—at least not with wheat bread. But if you do, I have no advice but to discard the sponge and start over, this time with a shorter cycle or a lower temperature.

There's a third smell you might run into: the alcohol smell of yeast. If you use baker's yeast often in your kitchen, there's likely to be a good deal of it hanging around—and some may find its way into your sponge. In fact, you might not need to add more yeast on your own!

Personally, I feel that any yeast growing in the sponge compromises the taste of the sourdough. Then again, if you're already using that much yeast in your kitchen, you may not mind the taste or find it a problem.

Visual. When sourdough bacteria are going full throttle, there's not a lot to see. It's only when the food supply runs low and they start spitting out carbon dioxide that you see signs of their presence. And it's only when they start dying off that they really roil the dough.

So, what you *don't* want to see is a mass of bubbles and foam in your sponge—or, in the later feeding cycles, any rising or "doming." If you do see such signs, it's either the bacteria dying off or contamination by yeast. At some point, you should be able to tell which by the smell, as I described above.

Gluten. While your sponge is fermenting, that's not the only thing it's doing. It's also developing gluten, the special proteins found especially in wheat. When wheat flour is mixed with water and allowed to sit, these proteins link together, forming a network that later traps carbon dioxide gas from your yeast, causing your bread to rise.

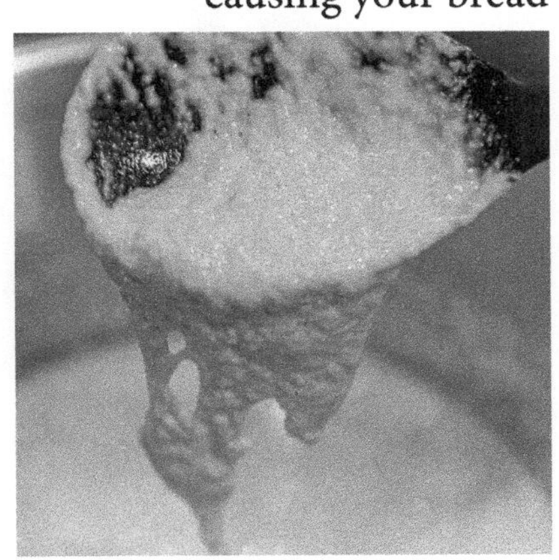

As you stir your sponge before its first feeding, the developed gluten should be obvious. Unlike when you first mixed the sponge, the mixture should be gloppy, with clumps hanging together, especially when you lift a spoonful and pour it back. And you should find this gluten network stronger at the end of each feeding cycle, till stirring the sponge becomes a bit of a slog.

It can happen, though, that stirring reveals your sponge to be completely runny, with *no* sign of gluten. This means the sponge has gone too long before feeding. The bacteria, running low on their preferred food, have turned to the gluten instead and devoured it.

Since you still have plenty of flour to add, an early loss of gluten is not a disaster—but it may still hurt the rise and make your bread denser. It may also increase the amount of extra flour you'll need to make your loaf. Again, shorten the cycle or lower the temperature the next time.

Temperature. If I could test my sourdough in just one way, it would be for temperature. This test gives you more specific, helpful information than any other test will.

The best time to check the temperature of your sponge is right before you feed it. That's because inserting the thermometer stem can carry surface microbes into the interior—and when the warm sponge is at its wettest, the growth of these harmful microbes can explode in less than an hour. Starting on a new feeding cycle right after testing will head this off.

To check the temperature, insert the stem of your folding thermometer at an angle, so the stem is nearly all submerged. Position the tip in the center of the bowl, near the bottom, where the sponge is warmest, but don't let it rest on the bowl itself, which may be hotter. You've already set up your warming device to heat water to 100°F (38°C)—so, you know that any sponge temperature *above* that is due to heat

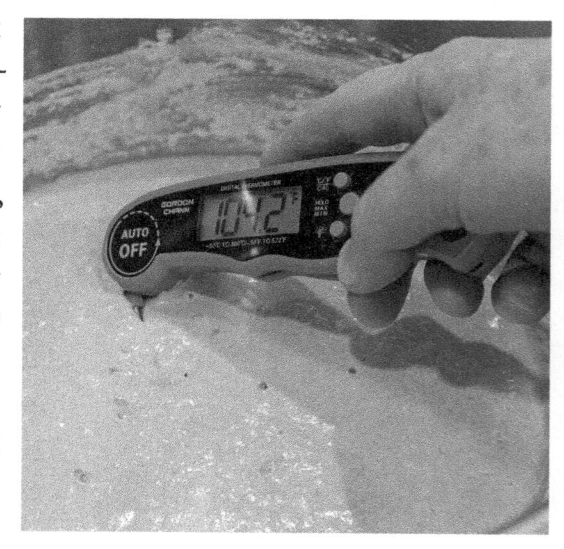

coming from the sourdough itself. (If this doesn't sound familiar, see the chapter "The Right Setup.")

Here are temperatures you might find, along with what they mean. (If you used a *different* target temperature for your device, you'll have to transpose these up or down, based on the difference.)

- Around 100°F (38°C). Fermenting hasn't started—or if you also see a lot of bubbles and froth, the microbes are already dead or dormant!
- Rising toward 105°F (about 40°C). It's starting to happen!
- Close to 105°F (about 40°C). Fermenting is zipping along nicely, with the feeding cycle at its peak of activity. You're on track for a nice, mild sourdough. (If you recall, this is the "optimum" sponge temperature I gave earlier in the book—the ideal *median*.)
- Rising toward 110°F (43°C). Food is running low, the microbes are stressed, and you're getting some extra sourness. You're headed toward a more tangy sourdough.
- Above 110°F (43°C). You're getting too close to running out of food. Next time, you should probably shorten the cycle or lower the temperature.
- Above 120°F (close to 50°C). Something is seriously wrong with your setup. You're cooking your sponge and killing your microbes.

With my recipe, I've aimed to bring the sponge between 105°F and 110°F (about 40°C and 43°C) by the end of each feeding cycle. But in some cycles, it just doesn't get that high—and that's okay. In the end, I still get great sourdough.

Besides testing your sponge, you can test the temperature of your loaf at the end of its rise. To keep from deflating the loaf, insert the thermometer stem at a steep angle, pushing the tip slowly toward the center bottom. Once you have your reading, pull the stem slowly back out, using your fingers to keep the dough from coming with it.

Look for a temperature right around 100°F (38°C)—the optimum temperature for the loaf. But a few degrees higher or lower is still fine.

Taste. The ultimate test. I often like to cut off a slice about an hour after the bread comes out of the oven. The next morning is a good time, too.

Depending on *everything*, the taste of your sourdough might be sweet, or tangy, or mildly sour. Whichever it is, it should be delicious—and ideally, you'll detect no bitterness or yeastiness or off-taste of any kind.

If you come *close* to that, your bread is a success.

Advanced Tests

Besides the tests you might do each time you make sourdough, there are others you might pull out for special occasions—whenever you feel that special need to immerse yourself in technical data, either to track a problem or to get a little reassurance.

Chlorine. If you're worried about chlorine in your water, you can use a "free chlorine" test strip to check how much is in there to start with and how much you're able to remove.

Water pH. A digital pH meter is very handy for testing acidity/alkalinity in water and other liquids. Though the meters normally come with calibration powders, I find it easier just to compare test results against known values—for instance, about 5.8 for distilled water, or 8.2 for my local water.

The meter's sensor needs to say moist, and it also needs to be rinsed clean with distilled or purified water after each use. I take care of both by keeping the meter standing in a cup with enough

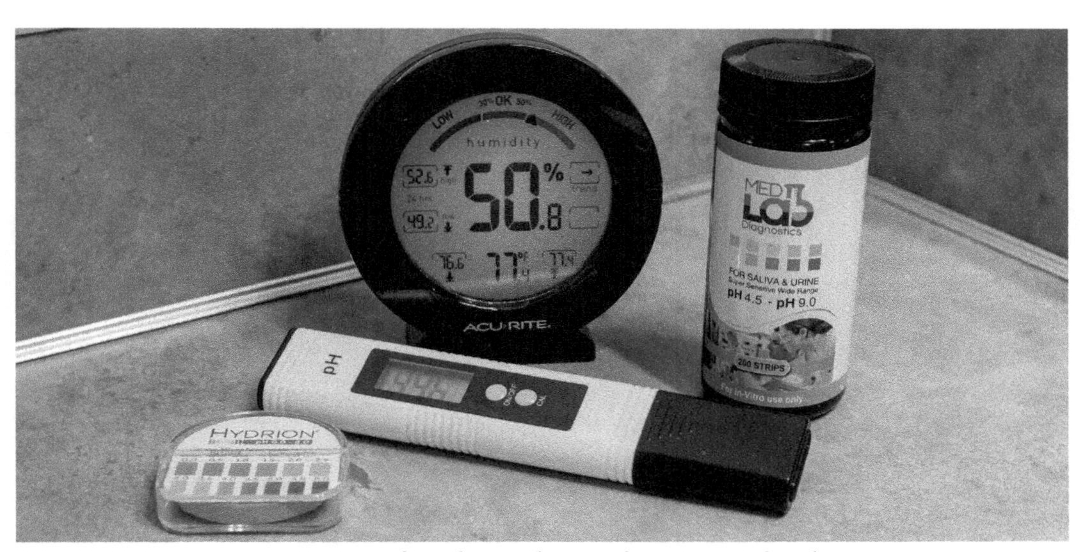

Equipment for advanced tests of smart sourdough

distilled or purified water to cover the sensor and swishing the end around in the cup after testing.

Dough pH. A digital pH meter won't work on dough, so for that, you'll have to resort to pH strips. (They're sometimes called *litmus strips*, but those are really something different.) You get your result by judging the color of the strip, so it's a pretty rough measure—but hey, that's fitting for sourdough, right?

At the end of a feeding cycle, pull out a tiny bit of your sponge or loaf and push one end of the strip into it, then compare the color you see to the chart that came with the strips. With each new cycle, the pH should drop—meaning acidity should have *increased*. To get sourdough's preservative power for fighting mold, you need a final pH around 4.5 or lower—which is about what you should get from my four-cycle recipes.

Test strips are made for a variety of pH ranges. You'll want a strip—or combination of strips—that covers at least the range 3 to 7.

Humidity. A digital hygrometer—humidity gauge—can help you fine-tune the amount of steam you generate to keep your loaf from crusting.

Scaling Your Sourdough

With most bread recipes, you can easily adjust for different loaf sizes or multiple loaves with simple multiplication, applying the same percentage to all ingredients. But with smart sourdough, the high temperatures complicate things.

In scaling my basic recipe either up or down, there are several special considerations:

- The extra water allowed for evaporation
- The differences in hydration caused by that extra water
- The heat retained by sponges of different sizes
- The capacity of your warming device

Let's look at some typical scalings to get an idea how these apply. (Note that my scaled variations are shown as recipe *sketches* rather than full recipes. Look back at the chapter "Making Smart Sourdough" if you need an explanation of those.)

Scaling Down

Nowadays, only "large" loaf pans are common—which is why the basic recipe I've given you is for a large loaf. Still, you might own a medium ("standard") or small pan and prefer that loaf size. In fact, I generally prefer the medium size myself, since at my age, the lower calorie count is welcome!

The recipe sketches shown here give scalings for two smaller loaves—a 75% scale to fit a medium loaf pan, and a 50% scale for a small loaf pan. (Since the relative proportions of the smaller pans are not exactly 75% and 50%, the unrisen dough will come up a little higher in these pans.)

Smart Sourdough (Medium Loaf)

50% WHOLE WHEAT—MEDIUM LOAF—4 CYCLES

9 ounces whole wheat flour, 9 ounces unbleached bread flour, extra flour for kneading, 2 cups water, 1½ teaspoons salt, ⅛ teaspoon yeast

Sponge: 9 ounces whole wheat flour, 2 cups water, 1½ teaspoons salt
Warm with a target of 100°F (38°C) for 9 hours.

1st Feeding: 3 ounces unbleached bread flour
Warm with a target of 100°F (38°C) for 3 hours.

2nd Feeding: 3 ounces unbleached bread flour
Warm with a target of 100°F (38°C) for 3 hours.

Loaf: 3 ounces unbleached bread flour, extra flour for kneading, ⅛ teaspoon yeast
Warm and steam with a target of 95°F (35°C) for about 3 hours.

Bake at 375°F (190°C) for 40 minutes from a cold oven.

The approximate final loaf weights of all three sizes are:

Large—2¼ pounds (about 1 kilogram)
Medium—1¾ pounds (about .8 kilogram)
Small—1¼ pounds (about .6 kilogram)

The scalings for the smaller sizes are pretty straightforward—till you come to the water. My basic recipe adds ½ cup water to allow for evaporation—and that's pretty much the same amount of evaporation you'd get from my recommended times and temperatures *regardless of recipe size*. So, our scaling has to factor that allowance *out*.

Here's the arithmetic in general terms:

Smart Sourdough (Small Loaf)

50% WHOLE WHEAT—SMALL LOAF—4 CYCLES

6 ounces whole wheat flour, 6 ounces unbleached bread flour, extra flour for kneading, 1½ cups water, 1 teaspoon salt, 1⁄16 teaspoon yeast

Sponge: 6 ounces whole wheat flour, 1½ cups water, 1 teaspoon salt
Warm with a target of 100°F (38°C) for 9 hours.

1st Feeding: 2 ounces unbleached bread flour
Warm with a target of 100°F (38°C) for 3 hours.

2nd Feeding: 2 ounces unbleached bread flour
Warm with a target of 100°F (38°C) for 3 hours.

Loaf: 2 ounces unbleached bread flour, extra flour for kneading, 1⁄16 teaspoon yeast
Warm and steam with a target of 95°F (35°C) for about 3 hours.

Bake at 375°F (190°C) for 35 minutes from a cold oven.

1. Subtract the amount of water allowed for evaporation.
2. Scale the remaining amount of water.
3. Add back the evaporation allowance.

For example, for the 75% scale of my basic recipe:

2½ cups – ½ cup × 75% + ½ cup = 2 cups

The water for the 50% scale is figured the same way, coming out to 1½ cups.

Since yeast amount is not critical, I don't bother scaling ⅛ teaspoon to 75%. For the 50% scale, though, you can eyeball the 1⁄16 teaspoon, or you can use a measuring spoon for a *pinch*—which is generally defined as that exact teaspoon amount. (And if you just can't help yourself, you *can* scale the ⅛ teaspoon to 75% with a pinch and a *smidgen*—1⁄32 teaspoon.)

Scaling Up

There are two likely reasons you might scale up the recipe. First, you might want to make two or more loaves at a time. Second, you might want to make a round loaf in a larger size.

Let's start by doubling my recipe to make two large loaves. Just as in scaling down for a smaller loaf size, doubling the recipe is straightforward for the ingredients *except* for the water, which needs evaporation factored out. The arithmetic here is basically the same and looks like this::

2½ cups – ½ cup × 200% + ½ cup = 4½ cups

The doubled mass of the sponge will retain more heat, raising the temperature as much as another five degrees Fahrenheit

Smart Sourdough (Double Large Loaf)

50% WHOLE WHEAT—DOUBLE LARGE LOAF—4 CYCLES

24 ounces whole wheat flour, 24 ounces unbleached bread flour, extra flour for kneading, 4½ cups water, 4 teaspoons salt, ¼ teaspoon yeast

Sponge: 24 ounces whole wheat flour, 4½ cups water, 4 teaspoons salt
Warm with a target of 100°F (38°C) for 9 hours.

1st Feeding: 8 ounces unbleached bread flour
Warm with a target of 100°F (38°C) for 3 hours.

2nd Feeding: 8 ounces unbleached bread flour
Warm with a target of 100°F (38°C) for 3 hours.

Loaf: 8 ounces unbleached bread flour, extra flour for kneading, ¼ teaspoon yeast
Warm and steam with a target of 95°F (35°C) for about 3 hours.

For two loaves, bake at 375°F (190°C) for 45 minutes from a cold oven.

Smart Sourdough (Double Medium Loaf)

50% WHOLE WHEAT—DOUBLE MEDIUM LOAF—4 CYCLES

18 ounces whole wheat flour, 18 ounces unbleached bread flour, extra flour for kneading, 3½ cups water, 3 teaspoons salt, ¼ teaspoon yeast

Sponge: 18 ounces whole wheat flour, 3½ cups water, 3 teaspoons salt
Warm with a target of 100°F (38°C) for 9 hours.

1st Feeding: 6 ounces unbleached bread flour
Warm with a target of 100°F (38°C) for 3 hours.

2nd Feeding: 6 ounces unbleached bread flour
Warm with a target of 100°F (38°C) for 3 hours.

Loaf: 6 ounces unbleached bread flour, extra flour for kneading, ¼ teaspoon yeast
Warm and steam with a target of 95°F (35°C) for about 3 hours.

For two loaves, bake at 375°F (190°C) for 40 minutes from a cold oven.

(three degrees Celsius). On the other hand, the sponge will take longer to warm up. On balance, then, you shouldn't have to change your temperature settings or the recipe times.

Your most likely bottleneck is your warming device. Though most setups can handle bigger sponges, fewer have room for two loaf pans.

To get around this, you could use *two* devices, or just a single larger one—such as the Brød & Taylor, which *does* hold two pans. (Since each loaf will be off center in that proofer, their temperature will be lower by about three degrees Fahrenheit—about two degrees Celsius—but that isn't enough to worry about.) Or you could

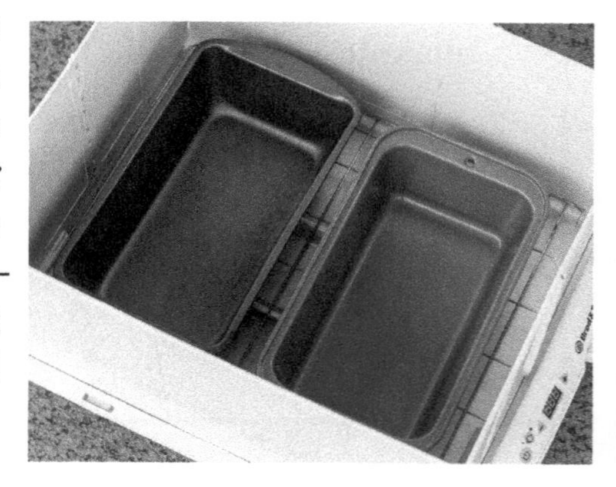

forget using a warming device for the loaves and just let them rise on your kitchen counter, perhaps with double the yeast to compensate for the lower temperature.

The recipe sketches here show scalings both for two large loaves and for two medium loaves. The same scalings can be used to make single round loaves in two larger sizes—but I can't offer reliable baking times for those, so be prepared to experiment, and keep your thermometer handy!

Limits to Scaling

In my testing, I've successfully scaled my basic recipe as far down as 50% and as far up as 200%. But I would be cautious about going much outside that range—that is, without adjusting other parts of the recipe.

On the bottom end of scaling, the problem is high hydration. Though you're reducing the amounts of both flour and water, the water reduction is not proportional, because the evaporation allowance doesn't change. The smaller the loaf, then, the higher the beginning ratio of water to flour. And with that higher hydration comes faster microbe growth and fermentation, making the microbes run out of food that much sooner.

The problem at the high end—along with the limited size of warming devices—is the way that larger sponges retain more heat. Enlarge the sponge too much, and temperatures will reach into that zone above 120°F (close to 50°C) where most microbes die off.

This is not to say you can't cross either scaling boundary. But the farther you go beyond, the more likely you'll need to adopt shorter feeding cycles and/or lower target temperatures to avoid failure.

Smart Sourdough (Triple Medium Loaf)

50% WHOLE WHEAT—TRIPLE MEDIUM LOAF—4 CYCLES

27 ounces whole wheat flour, 27 ounces unbleached bread flour,
extra flour for kneading, 5 cups water, 4½ teaspoons salt, ¼ teaspoon yeast

Sponge: 27 ounces whole wheat flour, 5 cups water, 4½ teaspoons salt
Warm with a target of 100°F (38°C) for 9 hours.

1st Feeding: 9 ounces unbleached bread flour
Warm with a target of 100°F (38°C) for 3 hours.

2nd Feeding: 9 ounces unbleached bread flour
Warm with a target of 100°F (38°C) for 3 hours.

Loaf: 9 ounces unbleached bread flour, extra flour for kneading, ¼ teaspoon yeast
Warm and steam with a target of 95°F (35°C) for about 3 hours.

For three loaves, bake at 375°F (190°C) for 40 minutes from a cold oven.

With all that said, I did once make three medium loaves—the absolute most you can fit in a Brød & Taylor proofer. (The water tray was shifted to the front to let the steam rise). So, I offer a final recipe sketch for that.

Customizing Your Sourdough

My basic sourdough recipe is designed to be as flexible as possible, allowing easy adjustment in a number of ways. We've already looked at scaling, but now let's look at other ways to modify it. (As in the chapter on scaling, I'll present each variation as a recipe sketch rather than as a full recipe.)

Wholeness

I find that 50% whole wheat gives a fine compromise between nutrition on one side and rise and texture on the other, while also

Smart Sourdough (100% Whole Wheat)

100% WHOLE WHEAT—LARGE LOAF—4 CYCLES

24 ounces whole wheat flour, extra flour for kneading, 2½ cups water, 2 teaspoons salt, ⅛ teaspoon yeast

Sponge: 12 ounces whole wheat flour, 2½ cups water, 2 teaspoons salt
Warm with a target of 100°F (38°C) for 9 hours.

1st Feeding: 4 ounces whole wheat flour
Warm with a target of 100°F (38°C) for 3 hours.

2nd Feeding: 4 ounces whole wheat flour
Warm with a target of 100°F (38°C) for 3 hours.

Loaf: 4 ounces whole wheat flour, extra flour for kneading, ⅛ teaspoon yeast
Warm and steam with a target of 95°F (35°C) for about 3 hours.

Bake at 375°F (190°C) for 45 minutes from a cold oven.

Smart Sourdough (25% Whole Wheat)

25% WHOLE WHEAT—LARGE LOAF—4 CYCLES

6 ounces whole wheat flour, 18 ounces unbleached bread flour,
extra flour for kneading, 2½ cups water, 2 teaspoons salt, ⅛ teaspoon yeast

Sponge: 6 ounces whole wheat flour, 6 ounces unbleached bread flour,
2½ cups water, 2 teaspoons salt
Warm with a target of 100°F (38°C) for 9 hours.

1st Feeding: 4 ounces unbleached bread flour
Warm with a target of 100°F (38°C) for 3 hours.

2nd Feeding: 4 ounces unbleached bread flour
Warm with a target of 100°F (38°C) for 3 hours.

Loaf: 4 ounces unbleached bread flour, extra flour for kneading, ⅛ teaspoon yeast
Warm and steam with a target of 95°F (35°C) for about 3 hours.

Bake at 375°F (190°C) for 45 minutes from a cold oven.

being simple to put together. That's why I recommend it for most bakers. Still, you may well prefer your bread more toward one end of the spectrum or the other.

The variation here for 100% whole wheat gives you double the vitamins and minerals of my basic recipe and has fine taste as well. Its main disadvantage—to some people, at least—is that it's denser, achieving only about a 50% rise. Also, slices may not hold together as well when the bread is a few days old.

My 25% whole wheat variation brings you more toward the "rustic" loaves made by artisan bakeries today. The whole wheat helps the fermenting and adds a bit of interest to the taste without dominating it or seriously limiting the rise.

Sourness

There are a number of ways to adjust the sourness of smart sourdough. Reducing the temperatures or the feeding cycle times will make the bread milder. Increasing them will make the bread more sour—though this comes with some risks. In the sponge, for example—especially early on, when the proportion of water is highest—your microbes can exhaust the food, causing a die-off. In the loaf, a higher temperature may impede the yeast.

One especially safe and effective change you can make is in the amount of yeast you add at the end. This shortens or lengthens the time needed for the rise, giving the bacteria more or less time to sour the dough in this final cycle.

Reducing the yeast by half, to 1⁄16 teaspoon (1 pinch), increases the rising time by around three-quarters of an hour. Doubling the yeast to ¼ teaspoon reduces rising time about the same. Note this is

Smart Sourdough (Less Sour)

50% WHOLE WHEAT—LARGE LOAF—3 CYCLES

12 ounces whole wheat flour, 12 ounces unbleached bread flour, extra flour for kneading, 2½ cups water, 2 teaspoons salt, ⅛ teaspoon yeast

Sponge: 12 ounces whole wheat flour, 2½ cups water, 2 teaspoons salt
Warm with a target of 100°F (38°C) for 9 hours.

1st Feeding: 6 ounces unbleached bread flour
Warm with a target of 100°F (38°C) for 3 hours.

Loaf: 6 ounces unbleached bread flour, extra flour for kneading, ⅛ teaspoon yeast
Warm and steam with a target of 95°F (35°C) for about 3 hours.

Bake at 375°F (190°C) for 45 minutes from a cold oven.

Smart Sourdough (More Sour)

50% WHOLE WHEAT—LARGE LOAF—5 CYCLES

12 ounces whole wheat flour, 12 ounces unbleached bread flour, extra flour for kneading, 2½ cups water, 2 teaspoons salt, ⅛ teaspoon yeast

Sponge: 12 ounces whole wheat flour, 2½ cups water, 2 teaspoons salt
Warm with a target of 100°F (38°C) for 9 hours.

1st Feeding: 3 ounces unbleached bread flour
Warm with a target of 100°F (38°C) for 3 hours.

2nd Feeding: 3 ounces unbleached bread flour
Warm with a target of 100°F (38°C) for 3 hours.

3rd Feeding: 3 ounces unbleached bread flour
Warm with a target of 100°F (38°C) for 3 hours.

Loaf: 3 ounces unbleached bread flour, extra flour for kneading, ⅛ teaspoon yeast
Warm and steam with a target of 95°F (35°C) for about 3 hours.

Bake at 375°F (190°C) for 45 minutes from a cold oven.

based on the *doubling time* of baker's yeast at the temperatures we're using. Rising time is *not* proportional to yeast amount!

My favorite way to adjust sourness, though, is to change the *number* of feeding cycles. Each cycle is a step up in sourness. Want your bread more sour? Add another feeding cycle! Want it milder, "sweeter"? Take one out! One of the beauties of smart sourdough is how easily you can make this adjustment.

As you've seen, my basic recipe includes four feeding cycles: the making of the sponge, the making of the loaf, plus two sponge feedings in between. But it can easily be adjusted to three cycles total, or five—and still always stay within 24 hours, if you don't count cooling time!

The recipe sketches here will show you how that looks. Note that adding a cycle adds three hours to the recipe time, while removing a cycle subtracts the same.

Mixing and Matching

One of the benefits of smart sourdough is you can easily mix and match different customizations and scalings—as well as completely different kinds of sourdough (coming soon)—to get just the sourdough you want.

Smart Sourdough (San Francisco Style)

25% WHITE WHOLE WHEAT—LARGE LOAF—5 CYCLES

6 ounces white whole wheat flour, 18 ounces unbleached bread flour, extra flour for kneading, 2½ cups water, 2 teaspoons salt, ⅛ teaspoon yeast

Sponge: 6 ounces white whole wheat flour, 6 ounces unbleached bread flour, 2½ cups water, 2 teaspoons salt
Warm with a target of 100°F (38°C) for 9 hours.

1st Feeding: 3 ounces unbleached bread flour
Warm with a target of 100°F (38°C) for 3 hours.

2nd Feeding: 3 ounces unbleached bread flour
Warm with a target of 100°F (38°C) for 3 hours.

3rd Feeding: 3 ounces unbleached bread flour
Warm with a target of 100°F (38°C) for 3 hours.

Loaf: 3 ounces unbleached bread flour, extra flour for kneading, ⅛ teaspoon yeast
Warm and steam with a target of 95°F (35°C) for about 3 hours.

Bake at 375°F (190°C) for 45 minutes from a cold oven.

For instance, what if you want a sourdough that's as close as possible to San Francisco style? To get that, you would merge the variations for "More Sour" and "25% Whole Wheat," while also making sure to use *white* whole wheat to minimize the whole wheat taste. The result should be pretty close to the San Francisco favorite. For your convenience, I've included the recipe sketch.

And finally, I offer a recipe sketch for the bread I usually make for myself and my wife, Anne—a 66% whole wheat in a medium-size loaf. Slice per slice, this gives you about equal the vitamins and minerals you'd get from my basic recipe for a large loaf but with only three-quarters of the calories. Great for old age and dieting! Be aware, though, that the slices don't hold together *quite* as well as with 50% whole wheat.

Smart Sourdough (Mark's Loaf)

66% WHITE WHOLE WHEAT—MEDIUM LOAF—4 CYCLES

12 ounces white whole wheat flour, 6 ounces unbleached bread flour, extra flour for kneading, 2 cups water, 1½ teaspoons salt, ⅛ teaspoon yeast

Sponge: 9 ounces white whole wheat flour, 2 cups water, 1½ teaspoons salt
Warm with a target of 100°F (38°C) for 9 hours.

1st Feeding: 3 ounces white whole wheat flour
Warm with a target of 100°F (38°C) for 3 hours.

2nd Feeding: 3 ounces unbleached bread flour
Warm with a target of 100°F (38°C) for 3 hours.

Loaf: 3 ounces unbleached bread flour, extra flour for kneading, ⅛ teaspoon yeast
Warm and steam with a target of 95°F (35°C) for about 3 hours.

Bake at 375°F (190°C) for 40 minutes from a cold oven.

Diversifying Your Sourdough

If you're like me, you may never tire of your basic wheat, water, and salt. But even then, you might find that a little variety in your sourdough can boost interest, appreciation, and delight.

Here, then, are a few more kinds of sourdough bread I've explored and recipes I've developed. All these recipes too follow the general instructions of my basic recipe and so are presented as recipe sketches, showing only changeable details.

All these recipes have their starting point in my 25% whole wheat variation. From there, I might change the whole grain, or add special ingredients at the end, or both, and then tweak other parts of the recipe as needed. (See this chapter's final section, "Designing Your Own," for more about these changes and adjustments.)

Important! When you add special ingredients at the end, they should go in *after* the yeast. That's to make sure the sponge is still warm and wet enough for the yeast to be quickly activated. Also, these special ingredients should be at room temperature, to avoid cooling the dough too much and slowing the rise.

Also important! As with whole wheat flour, avoid flour from *any* sprouted grain. The extra sugars in that grain will speed up fermenting and throw off my recipe times. And of course, you should also avoid flour from toasted or roasted grain, as it will carry no sourdough microbes.

Though any of these breads can be great in sandwiches, I generally make them as round loaves for variety. (For tips on that, see the next chapter, "Baking in the Round.")

Rye Sourdough

One simple way to vary your sourdough is to substitute another whole grain for some or all of the whole wheat. And the king of alternate grains is rye. My Smart Rye Sourdough was for a long time my wife's favorite among my breads—and it might still be mine.

Rye flour is notoriously sticky—and it can get a *lot* worse with overkneading, so definitely knead this dough by hand! The flour also tends to cause the sponge to form a heavy crust, but don't let that worry you. Just stir the crust into the rest of the sponge when you feed it, and the pieces will grow soft again.

Smart Rye Sourdough

25% RYE—LARGE LOAF—4 CYCLES

6 ounces rye flour, 18 ounces unbleached bread flour, extra flour for kneading, 2¼ cups water, 2 teaspoons salt, ⅛ teaspoon yeast, 2 teaspoons caraway seeds

Sponge: 6 ounces rye flour, 6 ounces unbleached bread flour, 2¼ cups water, 2 teaspoons salt
Warm with a target of 100°F (38°C) for 9 hours.

1st Feeding: 4 ounces unbleached bread flour
Warm with a target of 100°F (38°C) for 3 hours.

2nd Feeding: 4 ounces unbleached bread flour
Warm with a target of 100°F (38°C) for 3 hours.

Loaf: 4 ounces unbleached bread flour, extra flour for kneading, ⅛ teaspoon yeast, 2 teaspoons caraway seeds
Warm and steam with a target of 95°F (35°C) for about 3 hours.

Bake at 375°F (190°C) for 45 minutes from a cold oven.

Finally, be aware that some rye flour can smell less than pleasant when fermenting—especially if you grind your own—but this shouldn't affect taste.

Oddly enough, the wonderful, distinctive taste of a delicatessen ("deli") rye like this comes more from the caraway seeds than from the rye. So, it's important to use seeds that are *fresh*—not ones stuck in the back of your cupboard for years. When you open the container and first sniff the seeds, you should get a strong hit from them. (For older, weaker caraway, you can try increasing the amount—but it's not the same.)

Keep in mind that the oil in fresh caraway is potent. Don't add the seeds to your sourdough before making the loaf, because they could inhibit the growth of the bacteria. (In the baked bread, they could also cause tooth pain or sensitivity if they stay stuck too long between your teeth!)

When a loaf made entirely of wheat comes out of the oven, it's as digestible as it will ever be. But rye undergoes more changes as it cools, becoming more digestible over a period of hours. So, it's best to wait till the loaf is merely warm before cutting into it and sampling that wonderful taste.

Rye flour used in testing included Bob's Red Mill Organic Dark Rye Flour and my own homeground rye.

Deli rye like this is only the tip of the rye bread iceberg. If you're seriously interested in rye breads—and especially *sourdough* rye—see Stanley Ginsberg's *The Rye Baker*.

Buckwheat Sourdough

Another good grain to swap for whole wheat is buckwheat. (If you want to get technical, it's actually a *pseudocereal* rather than a true grain.) My Smart Buckwheat Sourdough lets the buckwheat

Smart Buckwheat Sourdough

25% BUCKWHEAT—LARGE LOAF—4 CYCLES

6 ounces buckwheat flour (not "light"), 18 ounces unbleached bread flour, extra flour for kneading, 2¼ cups water, 2 teaspoons salt, ⅛ teaspoon yeast

Sponge: 6 ounces buckwheat flour, 6 ounces unbleached bread flour, 2¼ cups water, 2 teaspoons salt
Warm with a target of 100°F (38°C) for 9 hours.

1st Feeding: 4 ounces unbleached bread flour
Warm with a target of 100°F (38°C) for 3 hours.

2nd Feeding: 4 ounces unbleached bread flour
Warm with a target of 100°F (38°C) for 3 hours.

Loaf: 4 ounces unbleached bread flour, extra flour for kneading, ⅛ teaspoon yeast
Warm and steam with a target of 95°F (35°C) for about 3 hours.

Bake at 375°F (190°C) for 45 minutes from a cold oven.

speak for itself, without any embellishment. Since buckwheat, like rye, is especially sticky, I reduce the water by ¼ cup.

Note that this recipe uses the kind of buckwheat flour most common in the United States, which is milled with the dark purplish hulls still on. That gives it a much stronger taste, as well as more sourdough microbes for fermenting. You can recognize this kind by the dark specks in the flour. By contrast, "light" buckwheat flour, often meant specially for pancakes or noodles, has a solid pale color and much milder taste—too mild for this recipe.

The buckwheat flour I favor is Arrowhead Mills Organic Buckwheat Flour. Another national brand gave me crust I considered too crunchy, possibly from *too much* of those hull bits.

Barley Sourdough

If mild flavor is what you prefer in sourdough—or what someone else in your family prefers—then barley's your grain. Replacing whole wheat with barley, with its subtle hint of sweetness, will bring you as close to a quality "white bread" taste as you can get in smart sourdough.

Of course, if that's not what you want, you might find my Smart Barley Sourdough a bit bland! But I do think it tastes especially good toasted.

For testing, I used Bob's Red Mill Barley Flour.

Smart Barley Sourdough

25% BARLEY—LARGE LOAF—4 CYCLES

6 ounces barley flour, 18 ounces unbleached bread flour, extra flour for kneading, 2½ cups water, 2 teaspoons salt, ⅛ teaspoon yeast

Sponge: 6 ounces barley flour, 6 ounces unbleached bread flour, 2½ cups water, 2 teaspoons salt
Warm with a target of 100°F (38°C) for 9 hours.

1st Feeding: 4 ounces unbleached bread flour
Warm with a target of 100°F (38°C) for 3 hours.

2nd Feeding: 4 ounces unbleached bread flour
Warm with a target of 100°F (38°C) for 3 hours.

Loaf: 4 ounces unbleached bread flour, extra flour for kneading, ⅛ teaspoon yeast
Warm and steam with a target of 95°F (35°C) for about 3 hours.

Bake at 375°F (190°C) for 45 minutes from a cold oven.

Pumpernickel

For centuries, the name *pumpernickel* has gone to particularly flavorful rye breads—usually sourdough—but its meaning has stretched quite a bit over time. I'm going to stretch it a bit more, to include bread from *any* grain with ingredients that are dark colored, nutrient rich, and strongly flavored.

Among those ingredients are the barley malt syrup, cocoa powder, coffee, and vanilla in my Smart Barley Pumpernickel. If you have trouble getting enough chocolate or coffee in your day,

Smart Barley Pumpernickel

25% BARLEY—LARGE LOAF—4 CYCLES

6 ounces barley flour, 18 ounces unbleached bread flour,
extra flour for kneading, 2½ cups water, 2 teaspoons salt, ⅛ teaspoon yeast,
4 tablespoons natural cocoa powder, 4 tablespoons barley malt syrup,
4 teaspoons espresso powder, 2 teaspoons vanilla extract

Sponge: 6 ounces barley flour, 6 ounces unbleached bread flour, 2½ cups water,
2 teaspoons salt
Warm with a target of 100°F (38°C) for 9 hours.

1st Feeding: 4 ounces unbleached bread flour
Warm with a target of 100°F (38°C) for 3 hours.

2nd Feeding: 4 ounces unbleached bread flour
Warm with a target of 100°F (38°C) for 3 hours.

Loaf: 4 ounces unbleached bread flour, extra flour for kneading, ⅛ teaspoon yeast,
4 tablespoons natural cocoa powder, 4 tablespoons barley malt syrup,
4 teaspoons espresso powder, 2 teaspoons vanilla extract
Warm and steam with a target of 95°F (35°C) for about 3 hours.

Bake at 375°F (190°C) for 45 minutes from a cold oven.

this bread could help you get your fix—and in the case of chocolate, without loading you up with sugar.

The bread may also serve to convince you that rye is not always even the best grain for pumpernickel. Barley, with less flavor of its own, lets the other flavors stand out more, for a taste that's more defined, less muddy.

Be sure to use *natural* cocoa powder—in other words, *not* Dutch process, or "Dutched"—because alkalizing destroys the extremely beneficial *flavonols*. (Most Dutch-process cocoa is labeled so, if only in small print. You can also check the ingredients list, which should show something like "cocoa processed with alkali." Or you can search or ask online about any particular brand.)

Espresso powder may also be called "instant espresso." But note that it's very different from regular instant coffee, which is made by drying brewed coffee. Espresso powder is instead made from coffee grounds.

If you like this bread's flavor but find it too strong—as my wife does—it's easy to moderate it. Just reduce the amounts of the four extra ingredients by a quarter, a half, or even three-quarters. (My wife loves the bread at half strength.) Of course, you can pump it up, too!

The barley flour used in testing was Bob's Red Mill Barley Flour. The malt syrup was Eden Organic Barley Malt Syrup. The cocoa was Hershey's Natural Unsweetened Cocoa Powder. The espresso powder was Medaglia d'Oro Instant Espresso Coffee.

Savory Sourdoughs

Smart sourdough provides a great setting for the flavors of many vegetables, herbs, and spices. There's really no end to the possibilities, so I offer just a few favorites as examples.

Smart Tomato Basil Sourdough

25% WHITE WHOLE WHEAT—LARGE LOAF—4 CYCLES

6 ounces white whole wheat flour, 18 ounces unbleached bread flour, extra flour for kneading, 2½ cups water, 2 teaspoons salt, ¼ teaspoon yeast, 1 cup chopped dried tomatoes in oil, 12 large sliced fresh basil leaves

Sponge: 6 ounces white whole wheat flour, 6 ounces unbleached bread flour, 2½ cups water, 2 teaspoons salt
Warm with a target of 100°F (38°C) for 9 hours.

1st Feeding: 4 ounces unbleached bread flour
Warm with a target of 100°F (38°C) for 3 hours.

2nd Feeding: 4 ounces unbleached bread flour
Warm with a target of 100°F (38°C) for 3 hours.

Loaf: 4 ounces unbleached bread flour, extra flour for kneading, ¼ teaspoon yeast, 1 cup chopped dried tomatoes in oil, 12 large sliced fresh basil leaves
Warm and steam with a target of 95°F (35°C) for about 3 hours.

Bake at 375°F (190°C) for 50 minutes from a cold oven.

Smart Tomato Basil Sourdough is my version of a favorite store-bought bread, the Sundried Tomato Bread of La Brea Bakery—a bread I sadly can't find where I now live. The dried tomatoes that my recipe calls for, often labeled "sun dried," are sold in small jars and packed with olive oil and herbs. The brand I've used is Mezzetta Sun-Ripened Dried Tomatoes. (Everything from Mezzetta is top notch.)

One small jar will give you the cup of tomatoes you need, or close enough. First drain the oil and save it for salad dressing, bread dipping, or anything else. Kitchen scissors are great for "chopping" oily foods. If the tomatoes have no salt or not enough, sprinkle on some yourself *before* adding them to your sourdough.

Smart Buckwheat Walnut Sourdough

25% BUCKWHEAT—LARGE LOAF—4 CYCLES

6 ounces buckwheat flour (not "light"), 18 ounces unbleached bread flour, extra flour for kneading, 2¼ cups water, 2 teaspoons salt, ¼ teaspoon yeast, 1 cup chopped walnuts

Sponge: 6 ounces buckwheat flour, 6 ounces unbleached bread flour, 2¼ cups water, 2 teaspoons salt
Warm with a target of 100°F (38°C) for 9 hours.

1st Feeding: 4 ounces unbleached bread flour
Warm with a target of 100°F (38°C) for 3 hours.

2nd Feeding: 4 ounces unbleached bread flour
Warm with a target of 100°F (38°C) for 3 hours.

Loaf: 4 ounces unbleached bread flour, extra flour for kneading, ¼ teaspoon yeast, 1 cup chopped walnuts
Warm and steam with a target of 95°F (35°C) for about 3 hours.

Bake at 375°F (190°C) for 50 minutes from a cold oven.

In my Smart Buckwheat Walnut Sourdough, I complement buckwheat's own nutty flavor with chopped walnuts. My wife's comment on this bread was that it was *too* good—in other words, it was hard to stop eating it. I had to agree.

Because of their high oil content, walnuts quickly go rancid and get bitter—so be sure to use fresh ones and to refrigerate what you don't use right away.

My Smart Mediterranean Sourdough is what I call a "regional bread," because it collects a number of flavors associated with a particular part of the world—in this case, Italy and Greece. It's tasty enough that my wife *insisted* I get the recipe into this book. (I should mention it's based partly on an "Italian" bread recipe of her own.)

The recipe's kalamata olives are something of a wild card, because they differ by brand. That's part of the fun! (But the ones I used were, again, from Mezzetta.) Buy them already sliced and then drain them well. A small jar of around 6 ounces should come close enough to the cup of olives I call for. If you're adventurous, you might try using the brine in place of some water in the recipe.

Smart Mediterranean Sourdough

25% WHITE WHOLE WHEAT—LARGE LOAF—4 CYCLES

6 ounces white whole wheat flour, 18 ounces unbleached bread flour, extra flour for kneading, 2¼ cups water, 2 teaspoons salt, ¼ teaspoon yeast, 2 teaspoons Italian herb seasoning, 1 teaspoon onion powder, 1 teaspoon garlic powder, 1 tablespoon grated Parmesan cheese, 1 cup sliced kalamata olives

Sponge: 6 ounces white whole wheat flour, 6 ounces unbleached bread flour, 2¼ cups water, 2 teaspoons salt
Warm with a target of 100°F (38°C) for 9 hours.

1st Feeding: 4 ounces unbleached bread flour
Warm with a target of 100°F (38°C) for 3 hours.

2nd Feeding: 4 ounces unbleached bread flour
Warm with a target of 100°F (38°C) for 3 hours.

Loaf: 4 ounces unbleached bread flour, extra flour for kneading, ¼ teaspoon yeast, 2 teaspoons Italian herb seasoning, 1 teaspoon onion powder, 1 teaspoon garlic powder, 1 tablespoon grated Parmesan cheese, 1 cup sliced kalamata olives
Warm and steam with a target of 95°F (35°C) for about 3 hours.

Bake at 375°F (190°C) for 50 minutes from a cold oven.

Smart Middle Eastern Sourdough

25% WHITE WHOLE WHEAT—LARGE LOAF—4 CYCLES

6 ounces white whole wheat flour, 18 ounces unbleached bread flour, extra flour for kneading, 2½ cups water, 2 teaspoons salt, ¼ teaspoon yeast, 1 tablespoon cumin, 1 tablespoon coriander, 2 cups chopped fresh curly parsley

Sponge: 6 ounces white whole wheat flour, 6 ounces unbleached bread flour, 2½ cups water, 2 teaspoons salt
Warm with a target of 100°F (38°C) for 9 hours.

1st Feeding: 4 ounces unbleached bread flour
Warm with a target of 100°F (38°C) for 3 hours.

2nd Feeding: 4 ounces unbleached bread flour
Warm with a target of 100°F (38°C) for 3 hours.

Loaf: 4 ounces unbleached bread flour, extra flour for kneading, ¼ teaspoon yeast, 1 tablespoon cumin, 1 tablespoon coriander, 2 cups chopped fresh curly parsley
Warm and steam with a target of 95°F (35°C) for about 3 hours.

Bake at 375°F (190°C) for 50 minutes from a cold oven.

Another regional bread is my Smart Middle Eastern Sourdough. It was inspired by my time working in a couple of falafel stands in Pacific Beach, California, back in the 1970s. Thank you, Rey!

Be sure to use *fresh* cumin and coriander for this recipe. Stale cumin is worse than useless. In one supermarket, I had better luck with cumin in a Mexican food section, as the turnover there was higher. (But that was in southern California.)

The parsley amount is just a rough guide. Chop the leaves—not the stems!—of a single bunch, and you should be fine. But do stick with fresh parsley, not dried flakes, and I recommend keeping it curly, not flat.

Sweet Sourdoughs

Sourdough sweet breads? Isn't that a contradiction in terms? Not at all, because the tang of sourdough adds a welcome counterpoint to conventional sweetness. Besides, haven't you ever had sweetened yogurt? If so, then you've already enjoyed a similar melding.

Sweetening sourdough, though, can be a challenge, because any kind of sugar is normally eaten by the sourdough microbes and turned to acid. But there is a solution: Add sugar that the microbes can't easily access. At least one way to do that is to add bits of sweet foods that won't dissolve or melt in the dough.

Smart Raisin Sourdough

25% WHITE WHOLE WHEAT—LARGE LOAF—4 CYCLES

6 ounces white whole wheat flour, 18 ounces unbleached bread flour, extra flour for kneading, 2½ cups water, 2 teaspoons salt, ¼ teaspoon yeast, 1 cup raisins

Sponge: 6 ounces white whole wheat flour, 6 ounces unbleached bread flour, 2½ cups water, 2 teaspoons salt
Warm with a target of 100°F (38°C) for 9 hours.

1st Feeding: 4 ounces unbleached bread flour
Warm with a target of 100°F (38°C) for 3 hours.

2nd Feeding: 4 ounces unbleached bread flour
Warm with a target of 100°F (38°C) for 3 hours.

Loaf: 4 ounces unbleached bread flour, extra flour for kneading, ¼ teaspoon yeast, 1 cup raisins
Warm and steam with a target of 95°F (35°C) for about 3 hours.

Bake at 375°F (190°C) for 50 minutes from a cold oven.

Smart Chocolate Cherry Sourdough

25% BARLEY—LARGE LOAF—4 CYCLES

6 ounces barley flour, 18 ounces unbleached bread flour,
extra flour for kneading, 2½ cups water, 2 teaspoons salt, ¼ teaspoon yeast,
4 tablespoons natural cocoa powder, 4 tablespoons barley malt syrup,
4 teaspoons espresso powder, 2 teaspoons vanilla extract, 1 cup dried cherries

Sponge: 6 ounces barley flour, 6 ounces unbleached bread flour, 2½ cups water,
2 teaspoons salt
Warm with a target of 100°F (38°C) for 9 hours.

1st Feeding: 4 ounces unbleached bread flour
Warm with a target of 100°F (38°C) for 3 hours.

2nd Feeding: 4 ounces unbleached bread flour
Warm with a target of 100°F (38°C) for 3 hours.

Loaf: 4 ounces unbleached bread flour, extra flour for kneading, ¼ teaspoon yeast,
4 tablespoons natural cocoa powder, 4 tablespoons barley malt syrup,
4 teaspoons espresso powder, 2 teaspoons vanilla extract, 1 cup dried cherries
Warm and steam with a target of 95°F (35°C) for about 3 hours.

Bake at 375°F (190°C) for 50 minutes from a cold oven.

That's the approach I've taken with my Smart Raisin Sourdough, which simply adds raisins to a straight 25% whole wheat sourdough. It's one of my simplest yet tastiest breads.

As you can imagine, this recipe lends itself to a great deal of variation. Just replace the raisins with the same amount of just about any chopped dried fruit—figs, dates, apricots, cherries, or even mixed fruit.

And things start *really* hopping when what you're adding to is a bread like my Smart Barley Pumpernickel. As just one particularly fine example, I offer my Smart Chocolate Cherry Sourdough. But as before, you can substitute about any dried fruit.

Designing Your Own Sourdough

As I mentioned, all the recipes in this chapter use as their starting point the 25% whole wheat variation of my basic recipe. (You can find that variation in the chapter "Customizing Your Sourdough.") With that as a template, you should find it easy to create new and unique breads of your own. Just do one or both of the following:

1. Replace the whole wheat flour with another grain that can supply the sourdough microbes—keeping in mind that the less refined and processed the grain, the more microbes it will contribute. (Think brown rice instead of white.) Or, if you want to stick with whole wheat, use *white* whole wheat to reduce flavor competition with your additions.
2. Add other ingredients to your sponge *after* the yeast—herbs, spices, seeds, nuts, vegetables, dried fruit, sprouts, whatever strikes your fancy. Don't forget that sugars in powders or liquids will be mostly consumed by the sourdough microbes, leaving little to sweeten the bread.

Depending on your changes, you might then want to adjust other parts of your recipe. For example, sticky or wet ingredients may require you to slightly reduce water. If your added ingredients are bulky enough to cool the loaf very much, doubling the yeast can hold down the rising time. Bread with bulky ingredients may also need a few more minutes to bake.

There's lots to explore! Have fun, and don't be afraid to try something really wild. (Did I tell you about my Buckwheat Coconut Brussels Sprout Sourdough?)

Baking in the Round

For day-to-day dining, you can't beat the practicality of a sandwich loaf. But making sourdough isn't always about practicality, is it?

Round loaves are great for when aesthetics are as important as taste—or sometimes, when you just want some variety. It's the shape I usually turn to for rye bread and other special treats—breads I'm less likely to make into sandwiches. And of course, it's the *only* shape for bread bowls.

The Baking Bowl Solution

There are several ways to make round loaves, including forming a boule to bake on a hot stone or in a cloche, or baking in a Dutch oven. Those options are presented well in other books and online, so I won't go into them here. Instead, I'll present an alternative that is simple, easy, convenient, safer than some other choices, and almost always overlooked: the stoneware baking bowl.

Made from unglazed stoneware, these bowls are shaped more or less like regular bowls but with added handles. For bread baking,

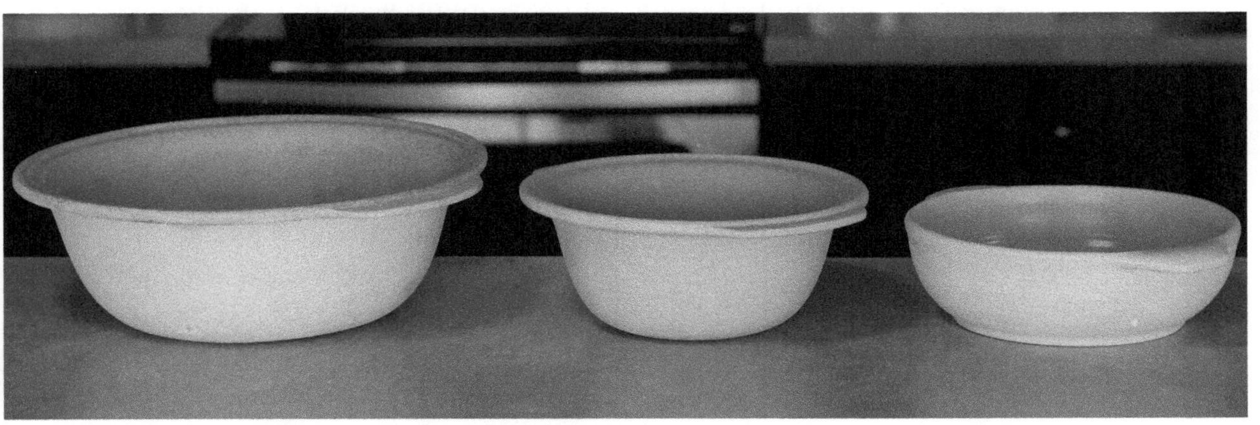

Stoneware baking bowls from Pampered Chef and King Arthur Baking Company (right)

they have two big advantages over most other round bakeware. First, they have rounded edges and sloping sides, for a more attractive loaf. And second, like cast iron, they can be seasoned, so that bread is not likely to stick.

Not many of these bowls are made today. But the King Arthur Baking Company sells one such bowl, custom made for them by Emerson Creek Pottery of Bedford, Virginia.

The King Arthur bowl has a broader base than most baking bowls, so that the shape is much like a casserole dish—and in fact, Emerson Creek Pottery sells their own casserole dish that's the very same bowl with a glaze. The size of the bowl is 8 inches wide and almost 3 inches high, with a volume that's just right for a large loaf—the loaf size made by most of the recipes in this book.

I found pre-seasoning to be essential with this bowl. No instructions for that came with the bowl itself, but King Arthur recommended this on their website:

1. Lightly coat the inside of the bowl with oil or vegetable shortening. (Don't overdo the oil, or you could get brown, gunky patches.)
2. Heat the bowl in your oven to 300°F (about 150°C) for an hour and a half. Things can get a bit smoky, so make sure you have good ventilation. (I would add, you might want to temporarily disable your smoke alarm!)
3. Once the bowl has cooled, wipe out any excess oil.

I followed these instructions using oil (not shortening), and after that, lightly oiled the bowl again before baking. The baked loaf fell right out. Though King Arthur supplied further tips to prevent sticking, I found the bowl didn't need them.

Another option you might consider is the stoneware baking bowls from Pampered Chef. The company no longer makes or sells them, but tons of used ones can be found online, often in great condition. The bowls come in two sizes useful for bread baking, Large and Mini.

The Pampered Chef bowls are a good deal heavier and clunkier than the King Arthur, but they have one clear advantage. Because of the gentle slope of their sides, each size bowl can be used to bake a wide range of loaf sizes. The Mini bowl—9 inches wide and almost 4 inches high—can handle any loaf size between small and large. The Large bowl—12 inches wide and a full 4 inches high—can handle oversize loaves like double medium, double large, and triple medium (as I termed them in my chapter "Scaling Your Sourdough").

These bowls gave me no trouble at all with sticking—all they needed was a light oiling before baking. But since I bought them used, I can't guarantee the same will be true for yours. Pampered Chef's online advice for these bowls does *not* include pre-seasoning, but it might not be a bad idea anyway.

Other Round Bakeware

The truth is, you can bake bread in almost anything that can go in a hot oven, if you find a size and shape you want. (Ever run across a recipe for Boston brown bread? It's traditionally made in a coffee can!) Keep in mind, though, that glazed or glass bakeware will likely give you more trouble with sticking.

For the large loaves made by most of this book's recipes, you'll want something that holds about 7 or 8 cups of water. For a medium loaf, that would be 5 or 6 cups. For a small loaf, 3 or 4 cups.

Round, glazed stoneware meant just for bread is available online under such names as *bread crock*, *bread pot*, or *bread baker*. (Don't confuse these with sourdough crocks, which often come up in the same searches but are meant only for storing starter.)

One good place to look is on Etsy. From the photos there, though, at least some were designed by people without much experience in baking.

If you just want a round shape and don't care much about aesthetics, the simplest, most practical choice is a cake pan. That's what I always used before discovering baking bowls, and I *still* use them sometimes. My go-to cake pan for a large loaf is 8 by 2 inches with a dark nonstick coating, from Chicago Metallic. The loaves it produces may not be worthy of photographing, but they taste great and bake without hassle, *never* sticking to the pan.

Tips for Round Baking

Here are some general tips for making bread in bowls and round pans.

- You might need to adjust—and maybe retest—your warming device setup for the loaf. (See the chapter "The Right Setup.") For instance, when warming bakeware with a broad, round base in the Brød & Taylor proofer, I need to place the water tray at the *front* of the heating plate—the same place it's kept when the proofer is stored—rather than in the center as usual. Otherwise, the bakeware catches too much steam underneath.
- Don't place unglazed stoneware directly on a glass stovetop or other polished surface. It will scratch! That goes also for a glazed piece with an unglazed base.
- The mass of a stoneware bowl will slow down warming and rising. To make up for this, you can preheat the bowl in a microwave before adding the loaf, aiming to get the bowl warm to the touch but not hot. You can also increase the yeast amount—to double, triple, or more.

• When oiling a bowl for baking, don't oil much higher up the sides than you expect the loaf to rise. Otherwise, you'll get a burnt, smoky smell from the exposed oil during baking. When in doubt how high to oil, aim lower, because the rising dough itself will push oil up the sides.

• Do *not* use spray oils on unglazed stoneware. They leave an undesirable residue.

• With glazed or glass bakeware, you will likely need extra measures to avoid sticking. Suggestions from the King Arthur website include using vegetable shortening instead of oil, sprinkling corn meal or semolina inside, or laying a circle of parchment paper in the bottom.

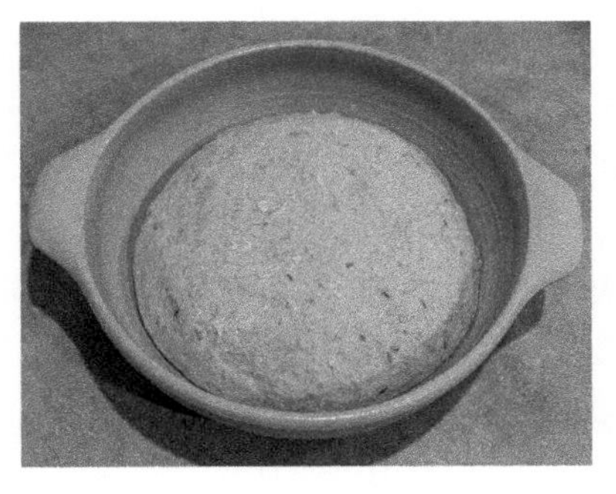

• Just place your ball of dough in the center of the oiled pan or bowl, seam side down, and let it spread by itself as it rises. If the loaf size is closely matched to the size of a pan or bowl, the loaf should reach the top at the peak of its rise. (That's not true, though, of bowls like the Pampered Chef that can handle a wide range of loaf sizes.)

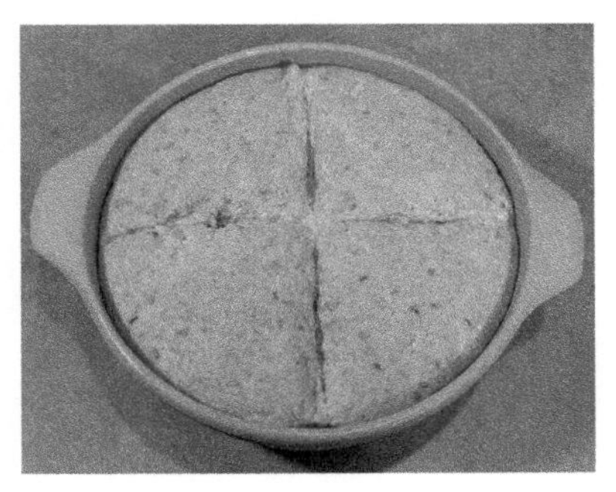

• Before baking, slash the top in at least two directions to allow expansion all ways. With unglazed stoneware, though, be careful to keep the knife point and edge from touching the bowl itself, which will quickly dull them.

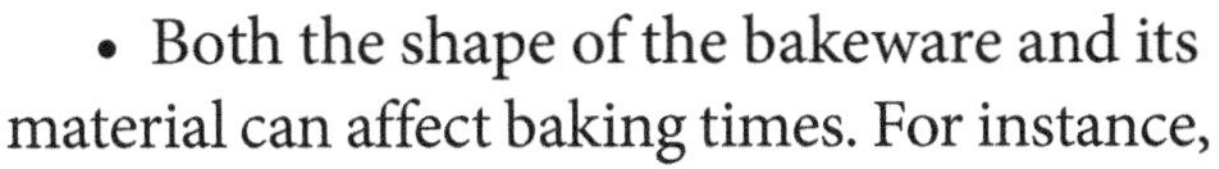

• Both the shape of the bakeware and its material can affect baking times. For instance, wide bakeware will catch more rising heat, while also forming a shallower loaf that heats more quickly. Stoneware will heat more slowly, needing more time in the oven. These factors can also affect *evenness* of baking, causing the top and bottom of the loaf to brown at different rates.

One way to adjust for all this is to bake on a lower or higher shelf—in other words, to set your bread a different distance from the bottom burner or heating element. Placing stoneware on a lower shelf, for instance, can give you a more properly browned bottom and keep baking time from getting so long.

• Unglazed stoneware is not meant to be thoroughly cleaned. Basically, you want the oil you apply to remain in a thin, baked-on layer so your bread won't stick. Soap may ruin this seasoning or leave a residue, so keep it away from your bowl. Also, the surface of these bowls is like fine sandpaper—you could sharpen knives on it—so avoid cleaning it with cloth, paper towels, scrubbing pads, or anything else that could leave fibers or particles. Best just to soak the bowl and clean it with your bare hands or a bowl scraper.

If you ever need to clean it more thoroughly, you can try using baking soda and a wet sponge. Some bakers say they've returned unglazed stoneware to a pristine condition by leaving it in an oven during self cleaning—though I doubt any stoneware is guaranteed for temperatures that high.

Making Sourdough Bread Bowls

If you've never eaten clam chowder from a sourdough bread bowl, you don't know what you've been missing!

I first encountered this treat while living around Monterey, California. It's a cultural institution there for restaurants to serve sourdough bread bowls filled with their house chowder made from locally caught clams—a delicious, hearty, satisfying meal all in itself, often costing just a few dollars.

Instantly, it became a favorite dish of mine. And I've looked for it in every other West Coast city I've lived in since—before finally learning to make my own. (Actually, I'm making the bowls, while my wife, Anne, is making the chowder.)

A bread bowl should be smaller than a normal loaf but taller and narrower—in other words, the size and shape of a soup bowl. And the best way to get that is to *bake* in a soup bowl! Modern ceramic and porcelain soup bowls are of course food safe, while most are oven safe too, and labeled as such on the bottom of the bowl.

But not *all* soup bowls are safe. For instance, if your bowl is very old, the glaze may contain lead. Others may be made in countries where safety has not been well regulated. If you have any doubt about the safety of a bowl at high temperature, *don't use it*.

Though a darker glaze may help a bit in releasing the bread, your loaf is likely to stick to *any* glazed bowl, even when oiled. The good news, though, is that the narrow base will mean less sticking at the bottom. To get out your baked loaf, you can hopefully just loosen it around the sides with a butter knife. Then again, you could just serve the bread bowl in the soup bowl!

For your recipe, I recommend my "San Francisco Style" variation, from the chapter "Customizing Your Sourdough." This will give you the most authentic taste, plus the reduced amount of whole grain will help the bowl hold together. If you don't want to deal with that recipe's five feeding cycles, you can just use the "25% Whole Wheat" variation, also in that chapter. Another great choice is my Smart Rye Sourdough, from the chapter "Diversifying Your Sourdough." Very nontraditional, but very delicious!

But what size recipe should you make? And what size soup bowl should you bake it in?

As a starting point, you'll get two bread bowls of big meal size by making a recipe for a large loaf—the size of almost all bread recipes in this book—and baking it in two 32-ounce soup bowls. For bread bowls of more modest size—the size shown in the photos here—make a recipe scaled down for a medium loaf and bake in two 24-ounce soup bowls. (For tips on scaling—and on warming multiple loaves—see the chapter "Scaling Your Sourdough.")

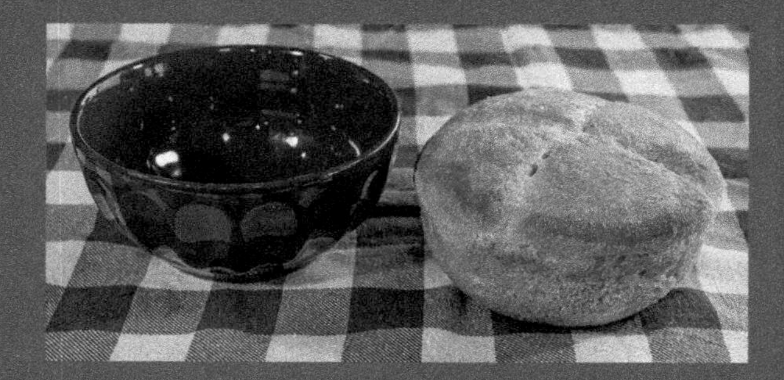

There are several things you can do to harden your crust so your bread bowls will better hold the chowder. (Just don't count on them being leakproof to the end!)

- Bake them longer.
- Bake them on a lower shelf.
- Bake them a few extra minutes outside of their soup bowls.
- Wrap them in cotton cloth only, not plastic.

One way to remove the loaf top is to cleanly slice it off with a serrated bread knife or other long, sharp knife. This way, you can use the top as a lid to cover the bowl again after filling it, or just serve the top on the side. Vivolo's, the Monterey restaurant where I first encountered these bread bowls, dipped the top's bready underside in melted garlic cheese and toasted it—an amazing treat of its own, especially if you dipped *that* into the chowder.

The other way is to cut a circle straight down through the top with a pointed, serrated paring knife or other sharp, pointed knife. You can then just pry off the top with your fingers. With this method, you get a stronger rim, making the bowl easier to handle and helping it hold its shape.

With the top off, you can go ahead and hollow the bowl in any way that works for you—with a spoon, a fork, your fingers, or any combination. A grapefruit spoon or melon baller is handy, if you have one. Just be careful not to pierce the bottom or sides or come too close to them.

For me, sourdough bread bowls are forever linked to clam chowder—but really, you can fill them with any thick, rich, chunky soup or stew. Whatever you choose, it goes in just before serving, so it will have less time to soak through.

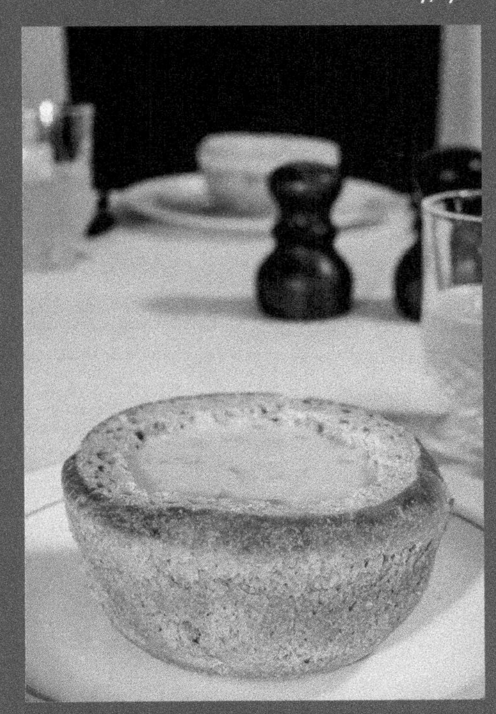

As for the etiquette in eating this dish, I'm afraid I never learned it and would probably ignore it if I had. I don't mind admitting that, after finishing the soup and scraping the inside walls with my spoon, I often tear the crust into pieces with my fingers and devour those too.

You'll have to excuse me now. It's New Year's Eve, and Anne will soon be serving her wonderful clam chowder in my first-ever sourdough bread bowls.

Grinding Your Own Flour

Nowadays, it's not that hard to buy whole wheat flour of high quality. I'm a big fan of the King Arthur brand, for example. Their White Whole Wheat Flour is what I used for most of my testing for this book, with wonderful results.

Still, with whole wheat, no big-name brand can ever be a match for what you can grind at home. That's not a knock of big-name flour. It's just the way whole wheat flour *is*.

You see, unlike white flour, whole wheat flour is perishable. It contains wheat germ oil, which soon goes rancid and becomes bitter. If you bought this oil on its own, it would come in an airtight container with all oxygen removed to keep it fresh, and you'd refrigerate it as soon as you opened it.

But when you buy whole wheat *flour*, it's sold just like its more popular, nutrient-stripped white cousin—in paper bags, stored, shipped, and shelved with no refrigeration. It has passed its prime long before it reaches you. And you can definitely taste the difference in your bread.

That's why I believe anyone serious about sourdough should consider grinding their own whole wheat. And it's why, as I finish this book, I'm returning to doing the same! (On the other hand, I'll keep blending my whole wheat with King Arthur's unbleached bread flour, which is *not* especially perishable and can't be duplicated at home.)

Choosing a Mill

Mills for home use come in two broad types. *Grain grinders* make flour by grinding grain between two artificial grinding stones or steel plates. They come in both manual and electric models—but unless baking is your substitute for a gym membership, I suggest you stick with the electric.

Impact mills, introduced more recently, throw the grain against steel posts or blades at high speed, and the impact pulverizes the grain into flour. Technically, impact mills don't "grind" grain at all, but I still use that term. Old habits die hard.

Nowadays, you can find affordable electric mills of both kinds that will do a good job for you. But both kinds have their own strengths and weaknesses. Let's look at some of those.

Noise and heat. The quality of an electric grain grinder depends largely on the strength of its motor. If the motor is underpowered, the grinder has to rotate the stones faster to make up for that. This makes the grinding extremely loud and—more important to the sourdough baker—it can easily heat the flour past the point at which sourdough microbes die.

On the other end of the spectrum is a grain grinder with a generous motor, such as my old Retsel or the newly popular Mockmill. This should keep your flour fairly cool—at least as long as you don't grind it too fine or in too large quantities.

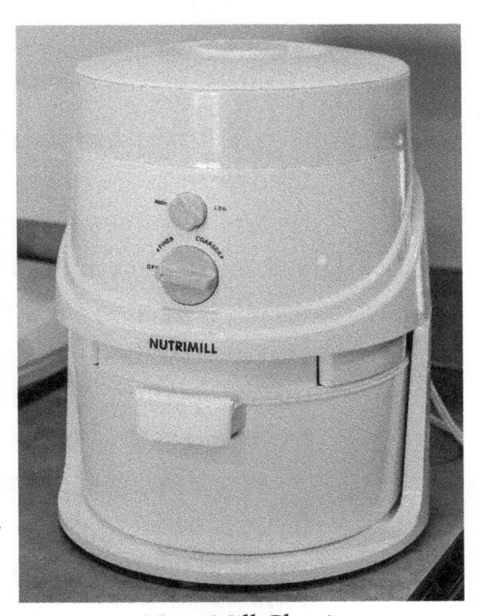

NutriMill Classic

Somewhere in the middle are the impact mills. The hottest I've measured flour from my NutriMill Classic is 118°F (about 48°C), which was when I was grinding a large quantity at a time. This is definitely too high for safety—especially since it may reflect even hotter temperatures at point of impact. But I find I can avoid the problem simply by refrigerating my grain beforehand.

Grit. The sad fact is that those two artificial stones in your grain grinder, when they're not grinding anything between them, are likely grinding each other instead. This results in grit in your flour, and that grit can gradually wear down tooth enamel. If you ever hear those stones scraping together, that grinder is placing your teeth in danger—a danger that never arises with an impact mill.

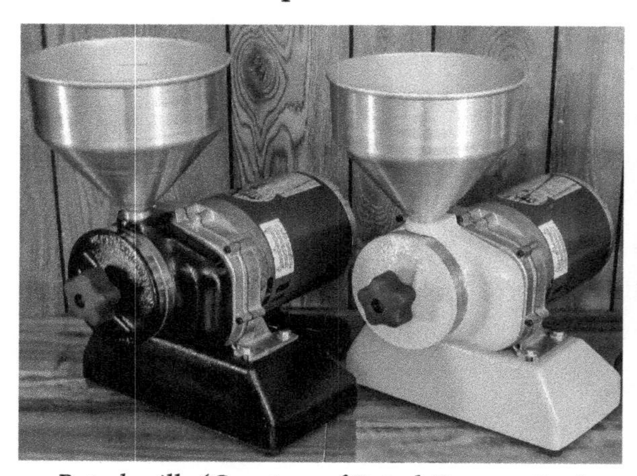
Retsel mills (Courtesy of Retsel Corporation)

Some older grain grinders, like the Retsel, let you replace the stones with steel plates—and I highly recommend you do that, if you can. Some newer, advanced grinders, like the Mockmill, have a mechanism that minimizes contact between the stones—but they cannot prevent it entirely, at least for finer settings, and what protection they do give relies on proper use.

Cleaning and maintenance. There's a small whirlwind generated within every impact mill, and if it finds the slightest gap or fissure, it blows flour through it. The problem becomes worse as connectors age and flour residue builds up, causing subtle misalignments. So an impact mill requires much more care in keeping parts clean and properly connected, as well as in cleaning around the mill after use. You may also need to clear flour from filters and traps in the flour bowl.

A grain grinder, on the other hand, just drops or shoots its flour into an open bowl or pan. Still, it could jam, or its stones could glaze, forcing you to take apart the grinder to fix things. This never happens with my NutriMill Classic!

Versatility. One disadvantage of an impact mill is it's really just for grain. On my NutriMill Classic, for example, beans such as chickpeas won't even fit through the inlet. And lentils disintegrate into a cloud of fine powder that escapes the mill and covers everything. A fine mess!

Compare that to my old Retsel, which used to grind both chickpeas and lentils for me, or the newer Mockmill, which grinds not only these pulses but also herbs and spices!

So, what kind of mill do I recommend? Grain grinder or impact mill? Personally, I'd start with an impact mill to grind grain with no danger of grit in the flour. But if I were using a lot of specialty flours, I might not mind having an advanced grain grinder as well, to grind what the impact mill couldn't handle. I'd be very careful, though, to prep the mill thoroughly and operate it so as to keep the grit to an absolute minimum.

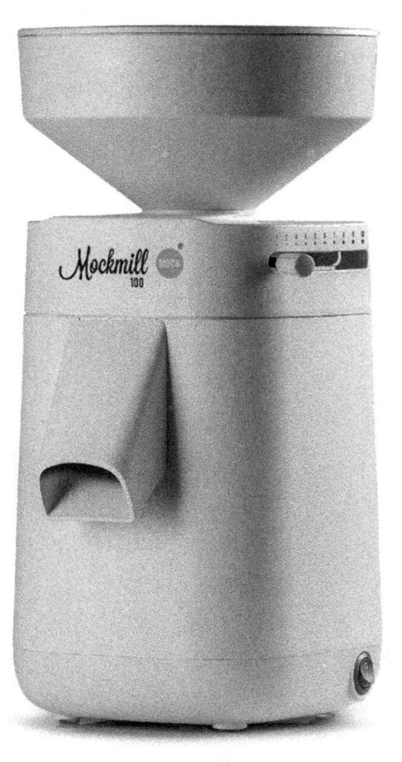

Mockmill 100
(Courtesy of Mockmill USA)

Buying Wheat

Wheat berries for grinding can be bought in the bulk sections of many grocery stores, health food stores, and co-ops. They can also be ordered in big bags or cans online (if you're willing to pay lots for shipping). But you have to know what you're buying. Only some varieties of wheat are suited to making bread, and some of those are better than others.

When I started making sourdough, I could buy berries of three wheat varieties.

Hard spring wheat. This is the kind found most often in bread flour (or *strong flour* in the United Kingdom). The *spring* in the name is for when it's planted. It's called *hard* because it's high in gluten—in fact, it has more gluten than any other wheat used for bread, allowing a higher rise. It's termed a "red" wheat because of the reddish pigment that darkens its bran coating and makes it slightly bitter. ("Red" wheat berries are actually reddish brown.)

The problem I found with hard spring wheat was that I was trading higher rise for taste. Frankly, the high gluten content could make bread taste like cardboard. And though souring could partly cover that up, it couldn't fully make up for it.

Soft winter wheat. This wheat is just about the opposite of hard spring wheat: It's planted in the fall, it's low in gluten, and it's a "white" wheat, lacking the bitter red pigment in the bran. ("White" wheat berries are actually golden brown.) The low gluten makes it useless for bread, but its lack of bitterness and general better taste suits it to pastry—and pastry flour is its main use.

Hard winter wheat. This is another wheat planted in the fall, but it lies between the other two kinds of wheat in both taste and hardness. It has less gluten than hard spring wheat, but still enough for bread. And though it's another "red" wheat with slight bitterness, it still beats hard spring wheat for fullness of taste. So, this was my original choice for sourdough.

Since those early days, though, I've found that another variety of wheat has become available—and it's better for bread than any of the others.

Hard white wheat. This can be either a spring or a winter wheat, but it's "white" instead of "red." It has plenty of gluten for bread and has better taste than either of the other hard wheats. Though still not as common in the United States as in other parts of the world, I think it's simply the best whole wheat for bread, and it's what I recommend, if you can get it.

Wheat Varieties

	HARD WHITE	HARD WINTER	HARD SPRING	SOFT WINTER
Color	White	Red	Red	White
Planting	Spring or fall	Fall	Spring	Fall
Gluten	High to highest	High	Highest	Low
Taste	Very good	Good	Bland	Very good
Bitterness	None	Some	Some	None
Use	Bread	Bread	Bread	Pastry

Buying Other Grains

Of course, wheat isn't the only kind of grain you might want to grind for your sourdough. Rye berries, for example, are another great candidate for home grinding. Though they're a bit harder to find than wheat, there's a bigger incentive, because rye flour goes rancid even more quickly than whole wheat flour! Also, commercial rye flour comes in different degrees of refinement, and if you grind your own, you can make sure you're getting the whole grain.

The truth is, it's often with more exotic flours that you get the most advantage from grinding your own—in freshness, control, and economy. In fact, some flours may be near impossible to get in any other way.

Whatever grain you're grinding, it should have *some* processing, just not very much. To be specific, you want the grain *hulled*—

in other words, you want it with its hulls *removed*. These hulls—also called husks or, collectively, *chaff*—are the indigestible and nonnutritive coats that protect the seed. *Unhulled* grain—with the hulls left *on*—has no place in bread. Luckily, it's not common to find unhulled grain sold as food, but it does happen. (By the way, *dehulled* means the same as *hulled* and the opposite of *unhulled*. Confusing, yes?)

What's left of the grain after hulling is called *berries* or *groats*—and these are ideal for grinding. At this point, you still have what's considered the whole grain, as it includes all nutritive parts of the seed. Any further processing, though, will remove nutrition or sourdough microbes or both. This is often obvious even in the lightened color of the grain. White rice, for instance, is little more than the starch that remains when you polish off the rice's dark coating.

For more help applying all this, let's look at barley and the several forms it comes in. First, you can buy unhulled barley—that's barley with the hulls still on. (Some people might want it, say, to add extra roughage to hot cereal.) Then you can buy barley groats or berries—barley with the hulls removed but the bran intact. Finally, you can buy *pearl barley*, with the hulls removed and some or all of the bran polished off. Obviously, hulled groats or berries are the barley to buy when grinding flour for sourdough.

Buckwheat, not being a true grain, is a special case. Though its dark purplish hulls when whole are too tough to chew, those hulls when ground up can contribute flavor and nutrition to flour—and microbes as well.

So, you have a choice. You can grind raw, hulled buckwheat groats for what's called "light" buckwheat flour, with its pale color, mild flavor, and fine texture. This kind is common, for instance, in France. Or for the kind of buckwheat flour standard in the

United States, you can grind buckwheat with the hulls still on, for a darker, speckled appearance, much stronger flavor, rougher texture, and more sourdough microbes.

While raw buckwheat groats can be found at online food retailers, natural foods stores, and even some supermarkets, unhulled buckwheat is sold mostly as seeds for planting—in which case, it's not meant for eating and may be treated with harmful chemicals. But you can also find it as seeds for home sprouting, and this should be safe for your flour. But check for that dark purplish color, as raw buckwheat groats too are sold for sprouting.

Besides milling, there are other types of processing that can affect a grain's usefulness in sourdough. You'll have to watch out for the following.

Sprouting. Grain is sometimes soaked for a number of hours and then dried again before packaging. This enhances its nutrition and converts some starch to sugar, making the grain easier to digest. If you make flour from it, though, the increased sugar will speed up fermenting and throw off my recipe times for feeding cycles. To keep those times reliable, avoid sprouted grains.

Toasting/roasting. Some groats are toasted for enhanced taste, easier digestion, and prolonged storage. For instance, it's common to toast buckwheat groats, which are often then called *kasha*. Though you can grind such groats for flour, all sourdough microbes will have died, so the flour won't help in fermenting.

Sad to say, it's not always clear from product names or package labeling whether groats are raw or toasted. For instance, Bob's Red Mill Organic Whole Grain Buckwheat is raw, but Arrowhead Mills Organic Buckwheat Groats are toasted. One clue is that toasted groats are darker. Customer reviews may also spill the beans—or rather, the groats.

Parboiling. In this process, rice kernels are partially cooked by boiling and then dried again, all *before* the husks and any bran are removed. This carries some of the nutrients inward in a kind of enrichment, and it also modifies the starches to need less cooking later. In the United States, parboiled rice has been popularized as "converted rice." ("Instant rice"—with brand names like Minute Rice and Ready Rice—is a whole different thing and not something you'll likely want to grind.)

Parboiled rice has its place, even as a flour—for instance, such flour is standard for making pancakes in India. But just like toasted grains, it's useless as a source of sourdough microbes, even when it's brown rice.

Using Your Mill

Here are just a few tips for making and using homeground flour.

- Keep all your sourdough bacteria alive and strong by avoiding high flour temperatures when grinding—preferably anything above 110°F (43°C). To be safe, *always* refrigerate your grain beforehand. You can also keep flour cooler by grinding smaller quantities at a time or by grinding at a coarser setting.
- Weigh the kernels, not the flour! If you're grinding only for immediate use, it's simpler to weigh the grain *before* you grind it, so you grind only what you need. (This is one of the advantages of measuring by weight instead of volume, since the volume can be measured only *after* grinding.) You won't likely lose much or any weight between hopper and bin—but if you're concerned, you can throw in an extra fraction of an ounce to be safe.
- If you're using artificial stones to grind oily non-grains like beans, the stones can get a slick coating that stops all grinding

till you take apart the mill and clean them. You can avoid this by mixing kernels of dried corn (maize in the United Kingdom) with the other food you're grinding. The ground particles from the corn kernel's hard surface act as an abrasive, scraping the stones clean as you grind, while the cornmeal you get is a fine addition to most recipes. For example, I used to grind flour for falafel patties in my Retsel from equal parts garbanzo beans, hard red wheat berries, and dried corn kernels. Rice might also work.

• Though an impact mill can make a fine, powdery mess when grinding pulses like lentils, it might handle them better if you mix them with grains. My NutriMill Classic, for instance, gives me little trouble when grinding a mixture of lentils and rice. If in doubt, though, you might run the mill in your kitchen sink, or even enclosed in a bag.

• Refrigerate any flour you won't use within a day or so. Put it in a tightly closed plastic bag or container to keep out moisture.

NutriMill Tips

The NutriMill Classic is not only one of the best home grain mills available, it's also one of the most popular. So, it's worth saying a few more words about it here.

The lid of the flour bowl has a rubber gasket that *must* be lubricated before you can get the lid on and off. But don't use oil! The way to do it is to dust the seal with flour. And since you don't want to do that each time, avoid cleaning the bowl with water between uses.

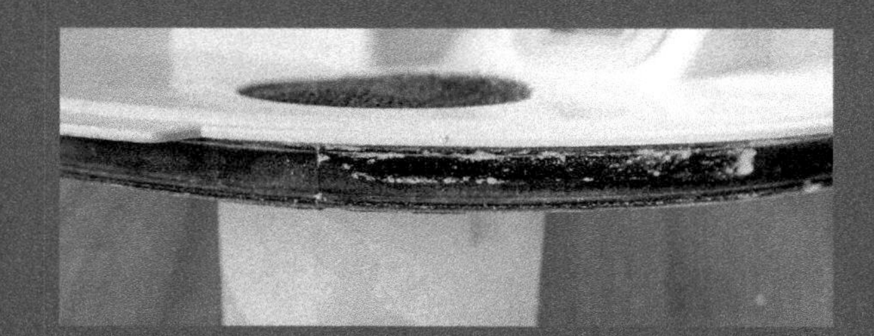

With this mill, the main thing to watch is the connection between the main body and the removable flour bowl. This connection is made by rubber grommets meeting to form what is theoretically an airtight seal. If the grommets aren't kept fairly clean and in good repair—or if they're not pressed tightly together—or if the bowl is pushed slightly out of position by flour buildup in the mill—you can get lots of flour shooting out onto your counter.

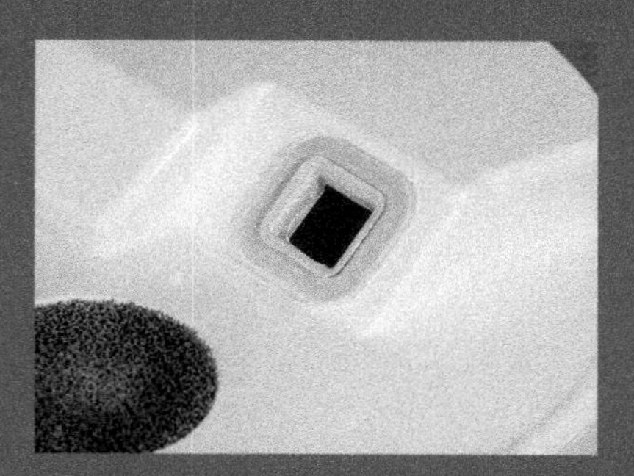

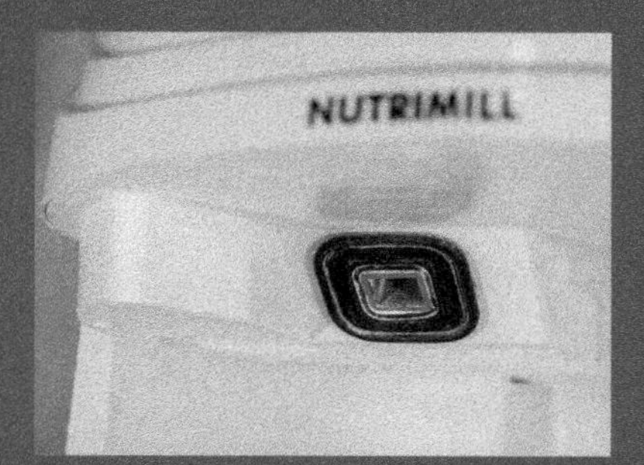

To help avoid this, I dry-wipe flour from both of the grommets and from the mill floor after each use. Also, during grinding, I hold the flour bowl tightly in place with a two-foot bungee cord encircling both mill and bowl. And I have spares of the bowl lid grommet, to replace that part when it wears out. (Of course, if you've operated this mill for a while without an airtight connection, the mill may need some major cleanup before the pieces can meet up properly.)

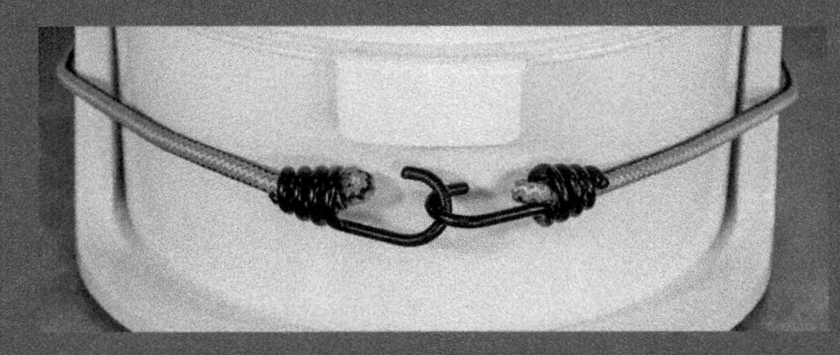

Other than that, the mill has required very little maintenance. I did manage to break one by turning it upside down—but it had already lasted for years, and its replacement has lasted even longer. (Don't ask me why I did that—I no longer have any idea!)

Also, I once had a handle crack on an aging flour bowl—due mostly to my habit of picking up the bowl by just one handle instead of two. I wish I could say I've learned my lesson!

Like many other home mills, the NutriMill Classic may heat the flour to the point of harming the sourdough bacteria. To prevent this, refrigerate your grain before grinding.

Making Sourdough Pizza

What would a sourdough book be without a chapter on pizza? Here's my humble contribution to the genre, once more applying the 24-hour, starter-free method of smart sourdough.

Making the Dough

My Smart Sourdough Pizza Dough is a basic dough you can use for almost any pizza. The recipe makes about 20 ounces, roughly enough for:

1 pizza at 16 inches
2 pizzas at 12 inches
3 pizzas at 10 inches
4 pizzas at 8 inches
5 pizzas at 6 inches

If you want more dough than that, see the chapter "Scaling Your Sourdough"—but I don't recommend trying to make *less*, since the recipe is already scaled down 50% from my basic bread recipe.

You'll notice this recipe uses unbleached all-purpose flour in place of the unbleached *bread* flour used in all of this book's regular bread recipes. (I used King Arthur Unbleached All-Purpose Flour for the testing.) I find that the reduced gluten makes the pizza dough more manageable, and I like the heavier crust it gives me. But feel free to stick with bread flour if you prefer, or to get higher gluten by replacing some of the all-purpose with semolina.

Not surprisingly, the final cycle of this recipe sketch is labeled "Dough" instead of "Loaf." At this point, you should add the yeast and knead the dough just as if making a loaf, only without shaping it and placing it in a pan. Then, since you won't need steam for the rise, I tell you to just leave the dough in a covered bowl at room temperature for this final cycle.

I've included a chart of sample schedules. If you're not ready to make your pizza when the dough is ready, just refrigerate it.

Smart Sourdough Pizza Dough

25% WHOLE WHEAT—20 OUNCES—4 CYCLES

3 ounces whole wheat flour, 9 ounces unbleached all-purpose flour, extra flour for kneading, 1½ cups water, 1 teaspoon salt, ⅛ teaspoon yeast

Sponge: 3 ounces whole wheat flour, 3 ounces unbleached all-purpose flour, 1½ cups water, 1 teaspoon salt
Warm with a target of 100°F (38°C) for 9 hours.

1st Feeding: 2 ounces unbleached all-purpose flour
Warm with a target of 100°F (38°C) for 3 hours.

2nd Feeding: 2 ounces unbleached all-purpose flour
Warm with a target of 100°F (38°C) for 3 hours.

Dough: 2 ounces unbleached all-purpose flour, extra flour for kneading, ⅛ teaspoon yeast
Leave the kneaded dough in a covered bowl at room temperature for about 3 hours.

Make into pizza at once, or cover tightly and refrigerate or freeze for later.

Pizza Sample Schedules

	"EARLY RISER"	"MIDDLE WAY"	"NIGHT OWL"
Prepare ingredients	7:00 p.m.	8:00 p.m.	10:00 p.m.
Make sponge	9:00 p.m.	10:00 p.m.	12:00 a.m.
Feed sponge (1)	6:00 a.m.	7:00 a.m.	9:00 a.m.
Feed sponge (2)	9:00 a.m.	10:00 a.m.	12:00 p.m.
Make dough	12:00 p.m.	1:00 p.m.	3:00 p.m.
Bake or refrigerate	3:00 p.m.	4:00 p.m.	6:00 p.m.

Making the Pizza

Chances are, you already have a favored way to make pizza, and chances are, too, it's more sophisticated than mine. But in case this is helpful, I offer my recipe for Mark's Sourdough Skillet Pizza.

Skillet pizza recipes have grown popular lately, but this is one with a difference: For safety, I do *not* put the skillet in the oven. The reason? When the skillet comes out, it's all too easy to forget that the handle is hot and grab hold of it! (And, no, a handle cover won't protect you long with a handle that hot.)

My goal with this recipe was to make a pizza that could be thrown together quickly for just one person—*and* be delicious. Once the dough is ready, you can make the pizza in a quarter of an hour.

The recipe calls for pizza sauce, but you really have a wide range of choices. Regular tomato sauce or pasta sauce will work, especially if you thicken it with tomato paste or cook it down. You could also try Alfredo sauce or even pesto. (My current favorite is Mezzetta Tomato Pesto.)

For cheese, grated mozzarella would be the traditional choice, but many cheeses could work well. Swiss is one of my favorites. But the most fun cheese I've tried is fresh mozzarella, which you can buy or even make at home. Starting with a consistency like that of thick tofu, a slice of it will melt quickly and become chewy. And if you have any of the fresh cheese left over, you can eat it as is, or maybe dip it first into balsamic vinegar or soy sauce.

Because the pizza is made entirely in a skillet, you can't really cook any extra toppings *with* it—but you can always add them at the end, either raw or precooked. Raw toppings might include fresh basil, olives, or red onion. Precooked toppings might include mushrooms, garlic, or red bell peppers, prepared by sautéing or roasting.

Mark's Sourdough Skillet Pizza

About 4 ounces Smart Sourdough Pizza Dough
Pizza sauce to taste
Sliced or grated cheese to taste
Raw or precooked toppings to taste (optional)
Olive oil or other vegetable oil

1. On a floured cutting board, flatten and spread the pizza dough with your fingers to form a rough circle about 6 inches (15 centimeters) in diameter. DO NOT KNEAD OR ROLL THE DOUGH. If needed, lift the circle by its edge and let it hang down to stretch it. If a hole appears, patch it with dough.
2. Lower the dough into an oiled nonstick skillet on medium-high heat. Cook uncovered till the dough is puffy on top and lightly browned in spots on the bottom.
3. Flip the dough over and cook uncovered till the original top too is lightly browned in spots. Press with a spatula to even the dough and to bring all points in contact with the skillet.
4. Flip the dough over again and immediately turn the heat down to medium-low. Quickly spread about a teaspoon of oil on top, then the sauce, then the cheese.
5. Cover the skillet. Taking care not to burn the crust, cook till the cheese is nearly all melted.
6. Remove the skillet from the heat, remove the pizza, and place it on a cooling rack. Add any raw or precooked toppings to the pizza and let it cool for a couple of minutes or so.
7. Cut the pizza into thirds or quarters and serve.

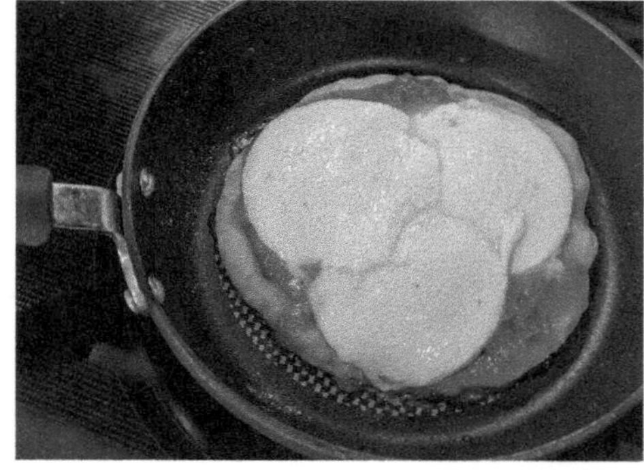

Making Sourdough Pancakes

With traditional sourdough, making sourdough pancakes is little more than an afterthought—just a way to use up "discards" from starter feedings. But with smart sourdough, it's a door to a whole new world of taste treats. Just as with bread dough, you can develop any of a wide variety of sourdough batters from scratch in less than 24 hours.

Oddly enough, in the United States, sourdough pancakes are not even meant to be sour. Instead, the acid in the batter is supposed to use itself up in reacting with baking soda (bicarbonate of soda) and creating enough carbon dioxide for a quick rise and a light texture.

But forget that! In these recipes, we'll aim to keep all the lactic and acetic acid we can produce. That's where the taste is!

The basic method is the same you used to ferment a sponge for bread—so I again present my recipes as recipe sketches. Of course, there's no "Loaf" cycle, and you'll note that "Sponge" has changed to "Batter," since the sponge simply *becomes* the batter as you keep feeding it, with no dividing line. For your warming device, you'll need only your sponge setup throughout.

With pancakes, we're dealing with a much higher ratio of water to flour than with bread—in my recipes, about double—and this greatly speeds up the fermenting. To deal with this, we need a lower target temperature and fewer feeding cycles. These recipes all call for three cycles at a target of 90°F (32°C).

You'll recall that our target for a bread loaf was a few degrees higher than this—95°F (35°C). With pancake batter, though, we're not adding steam, which by itself raised the temperature a few

Pancake Setup Temperatures

	OPTIMUM	TARGET
Batter	95°F (35°C)	90°F (32°C)

degrees. So, for this lower target with *no* steam, it *might* work to use the exact same temperature setting on your warming device that you used for a loaf.

To check that, test for this new target as detailed in the chapter "The Right Setup," following the instructions for a sponge. Here, though, are recommended settings for the three sample devices featured earlier, as tested with a stainless steel mixing bowl.

Brød & Taylor proofer: For the second generation, set the temperature to 95°F (35°C) in Proofer Mode. For the first generation—with no separate modes—set it to 90°F (32°C).

Instant Pot: Keep Warm Less (Some models do not offer this setting. You can instead try Keep Warm Normal with your bowl lifted higher above the pot.)

Sous vide cooker: 90°F (32°C)

As with bread, settings for our target temperature are meant to bring our sourdough batter to an *optimum* temperature that's a few degrees higher, once the sourdough adds the heat of its own activity. For pancakes, I've figured that optimum to be 95°F (35°C). If you're testing the temperature of your batter, then, your readings should normally be within a few degrees higher or lower than that optimum.

A few general tips for making these recipes:

• When buying ingredients, don't forget my earlier warnings against flour from sprouted or toasted grain. In fact, you should extend that to sprouted or toasted *anything* that's added at the end.

• With such high hydration, you'll likely get lumps of flour in your batter, at least at first. You can easily beat them out with a whisk.

• To thin a pancake after pouring the batter, you can spread it with the back of your spoon or ladle.

Here again, I include a chart with sample schedules. Rather than try to time the batter for a meal, I suggest you refrigerate the batter at the end of its feeding cycles, then take it out whenever you're ready to cook.

Pancake Sample Schedules

	"EARLY RISER"	"MIDDLE WAY"	"NIGHT OWL"
Prepare ingredients	7:00 p.m.	8:00 p.m.	10:00 p.m.
Make batter	9:00 p.m.	10:00 p.m.	12:00 a.m.
Feed batter (1)	6:00 a.m.	7:00 a.m.	9:00 a.m.
Feed batter (2)	9:00 a.m.	10:00 a.m.	12:00 p.m.
Cook or refrigerate	12:00 p.m.	1:00 p.m.	3:00 p.m.

Unleavened Pancakes

Though Americans generally like their pancakes fluffy, many pancakes of the world use no leavening at all. It's in that vein I offer my Smart Sourdough No-Rise Pancakes. Just as our basic bread recipe had a bare minimum of ingredients, this basic pancake recipe has even fewer—just wheat, water, and salt!

But don't worry. With its sourdough tang, this pancake is still quite tasty when eaten with a favorite syrup or other topping or even on its own. Whenever my mother visited, I could count on her asking me to make her this kind of pancake.

The recipe makes three cups of batter, roughly enough for:

18 pancakes at 4 inches
12 pancakes at 5 inches
9 pancakes at 6 inches

If you want to scale the recipe for more or less batter, remember you'll have to take account of the water allowed for evaporation. (For a reminder, see the chapter "Scaling Your Sourdough.") In this recipe, though, the reduced temperature and time mean the evaporation allowance is also reduced—to just ¼ cup. So, for example, the calculation for water in a half batch would be:

2¼ cups – ¼ cup × 50% + ¼ cup = 1¼ cups

It's fine to scale this recipe down to 50%—but as with my bread, I can't guarantee anything below that. I imagine you can also scale up to at least 200% and probably much higher—but never having had to feed that many people, I can't say I've tried it!

Like my basic bread recipe, this basic pancake recipe is easy to customize. You can use whole wheat flour in any percentage ranging from 25% to 100%. You can adjust sourness by adding or subtracting a feeding cycle. And you can thin or thicken the batter by adding extra water or flour at the end.

Smart Sourdough No-Rise Pancakes

50% WHOLE WHEAT—3 CUPS—3 CYCLES

6 ounces whole wheat flour, 6 ounces unbleached bread flour, 2¼ cups water, 1½ teaspoons salt

Batter: 6 ounces whole wheat flour, 2¼ cups water, 1½ teaspoons salt
Warm with a target of 90°F (32°C) for 9 hours.

1st Feeding: 3 ounces unbleached bread flour
Warm with a target of 90°F (32°C) for 3 hours.

2nd Feeding: 3 ounces unbleached bread flour
Warm with a target of 90°F (32°C) for 3 hours.

Thicken or thin to taste, then cook at once in an oiled nonstick skillet or refrigerate for later.

You can also explore different tastes by substituting different flours for the whole wheat—as long as at least half the flour in the initial mix of the batter is whole grain. We'll look at some special variations shortly.

Leavened Pancakes

Once you have a basic sourdough pancake batter, it's easy to add ingredients to get a full rise. The recipe sketch for Smart Sourdough Malt Pancakes shows my favorite additions, which go in only when the fermenting is done.

Since the batter's initial mix already contributes all needed liquid, the milk I add at the end is not whole but powdered—the standard amount of powder for the amount of water left in the batter after expected evaporation.

Smart Sourdough Malt Pancakes

50% WHOLE WHEAT—4 CUPS—3 CYCLES

6 ounces whole wheat flour, 6 ounces unbleached bread flour, 2¼ cups water, 1½ teaspoons salt, 6 tablespoons powdered milk, 4 tablespoons barley malt syrup, 1 tablespoon vegetable oil, 1 teaspoon double-acting baking powder, 2 beaten eggs

Batter: 6 ounces whole wheat flour, 2¼ cups water, 1½ teaspoons salt
Warm with a target of 90°F (32°C) for 9 hours.

1st Feeding: 3 ounces unbleached bread flour
Warm with a target of 90°F (32°C) for 3 hours.

2nd Feeding: 3 ounces unbleached bread flour
Warm with a target of 90°F (32°C) for 3 hours.

Additions: 6 tablespoons powdered milk, 4 tablespoons barley malt syrup, 1 tablespoon vegetable oil, 1 teaspoon double-acting baking powder, 2 beaten eggs

Thicken or thin to taste, then cook at once in an oiled nonstick skillet or refrigerate for later.

As a special treat, I replace the typical white sugar with barley malt syrup. That's what really makes this pancake, but if it's not a convenient choice, you can try substituting the same amount of good-quality honey. I tested with Eden Organic Barley Malt Syrup.

With the additions, you get about four cups of batter, roughly enough for:

24 pancakes at 4 inches
16 pancakes at 5 inches
12 pancakes at 6 inches

Buckwheat Pancakes

Spoiler alert! I don't think there's a tastier recipe in this book than the one given here—or a simpler one, either. If you make no other pancake in this chapter, don't skip this one!

Traditionally, buckwheat was grown and eaten where the soil wasn't fertile enough for wheat. Nowadays, of course, you can easily get wheat almost anywhere, but buckwheat lives on in many regional cuisines. And that's no doubt in part due to its popularity in buckwheat pancakes.

Probably the most famous of these are the unleavened *galettes de sarrasin* (literally, "buckwheat pancakes") of the Brittany region of France. From that part of the world, they migrated with the French Acadians to eastern Canada, where the pancakes were called *ployes*, and then on to Louisiana (where *Acadian* became "Cajun"). Though the recipes you now find for these French-style pancakes seldom include fermenting, that's traditionally how they're made.

Buckwheat pancakes have something of a split personality, because there are two distinct kinds of buckwheat flour. In the native regions of the French buckwheat pancake and its descendants, you have what's called "light" buckwheat flour, milled from buckwheat after its dark purplish hulls have been removed. With this pale, fine flour, you can make your pancakes entirely from buckwheat, or pretty close.

In other places, such as most of the United States, buckwheat flour is milled with the hulls still on—as you can see by the dark flecks in the flour. This flour has a much stronger taste and holds together less well. So, to use it in pancakes, you cut back the amount of buckwheat and use wheat for the rest.

This more common, speckled kind of buckwheat flour is what I use for my Smart Sourdough Buckwheat Pancakes. The buckwheat

Smart Sourdough Buckwheat Pancakes

25% BUCKWHEAT—3 CUPS—3 CYCLES

3 ounces buckwheat flour (not "light"), 9 ounces unbleached all-purpose flour, 2½ cups water, 1½ teaspoons salt

Batter: 3 ounces buckwheat flour, 3 ounces unbleached all-purpose flour,
2½ cups water, 1½ teaspoons salt
Warm with a target of 90°F (32°C) for 9 hours.

1st Feeding: 3 ounces unbleached all-purpose flour
Warm with a target of 90°F (32°C) for 3 hours.

2nd Feeding: 3 ounces unbleached all-purpose flour
Warm with a target of 90°F (32°C) for 3 hours.

Thicken or thin to taste, then cook at once in an oiled nonstick skillet or refrigerate for later.

is limited to 25%, which is still plenty strong! Because of buckwheat's stickiness, I add a bit extra water and switch to unbleached all-purpose flour from my usual unbleached bread flour.

The buckwheat flour I used for testing was Arrowhead Mills Organic Buckwheat Flour. If you'd like to try grinding your own, see my tips on buying buckwheat in the chapter "Grinding Your Own Flour."

Search online for "sweet savory galettes" for many ways to enjoy buckwheat pancakes. One popular yet super simple way is folded over melted cheese—and in fact, this is how I first tasted them, during the Festival of Saint Joseph in 1979 at France's Community of the Ark. Once the pancake is cooked on both sides, flip it over once more in the skillet, sprinkle it with grated cheese—Swiss is my favorite for that—then fold the pancake over and serve.

Rice Pancakes

Rice too can be made into pancakes with the help of something to hold it together. My recipe for Smart Sourdough Rice Pancakes is a simple example, combining white rice flour with some brown rice flour to stoke the ferment, plus a little wheat flour as a binder. This mild, unleavened pancake tastes great with maple syrup. My favored rice flours for it are Arrowhead Mills Organic White Rice Flour and Arrowhead Mills Organic Brown Rice Flour.

In much of South and Southeast Asia, rice supplants wheat as the dominant grain. So, in this region, you'd expect there to be a rich variety of rice pancakes—and there is!

In the traditional absence of wheat and its gluten, most of these pancakes have needed a different binder to hold them

Smart Sourdough Rice Pancakes

25% BROWN RICE—50% WHITE RICE—3 CUPS—3 CYCLES

3 ounces brown rice flour, 6 ounces white rice flour,
3 ounces unbleached bread flour, 2¼ cups water, 1½ teaspoons salt

Batter: 3 ounces brown rice flour, 3 ounces white rice flour, 2¼ cups water, 1½ teaspoons salt
Warm with a target of 90°F (32°C) for 9 hours.

1st Feeding: 3 ounces white rice flour
Warm with a target of 90°F (32°C) for 3 hours.

2nd Feeding: 3 ounces unbleached bread flour
Warm with a target of 90°F (32°C) for 3 hours.

Thicken or thin to taste, then cook at once in an oiled nonstick skillet or refrigerate for later.

together—and in the vegetarianism practiced by Hindus, eggs are forbidden, too! Often, then, the binder has come from *pulses*, a family of high-protein foods that includes beans, peas, and lentils.

The most famous rice pancake is south India's *dosa*, which I personally grew addicted to on a visit there in 1978. Dosa are traditionally cooked from fermented batter and served wrapped around hearty fillings. Home cooks today usually make them by soaking, wet-grinding, and then fermenting rice and pulses. But my Smart Dosa recipe uses both rice and pulse as flour instead—an approach that Indian cooks themselves often say is more convenient, and that may be more traditional as well.

I'll be straight with you: I was unable to find any commercial, easily obtainable flours in the United States that gave me a decent dosa. My Smart Dosa recipe, then, is meant only for those who can grind their own flour. Yes, that's one more reason to own a mill!

Also, my recipe takes advantage of the latitude in the term *dosa*—which in India has as broad a meaning as our word *pancake*—to prioritize sourness and convenience over texture and cultural authenticity. That means I've replaced the most common Indian duo of *urad dal* and *idli* rice with the American team of lentils and regular short or medium grain white rice, with some brown thrown in for the ferment. May Vishnu forgive me. (And if He could taste this, I think He would.)

Lentils can be a challenge to grind. With a grain grinder, their oiliness can give you glazed stones, while in an impact mill, their hardness can produce a fine, powdery mess. What will help in either case is to measure out your lentils and rice and then mix them together *before* grinding. When ground with the lentils, the rice helps keep grinding stones clean and, in an impact mill, holds down fine powder. My recipe encourages this joint grinding by calling for "blended flours."

Smart Dosa

25% LENTIL—25% BROWN RICE—50% WHITE RICE—3 CUPS—3 CYCLES

12 ounces blended flours (3 ounces lentil, 3 ounces short or medium grain brown rice, 6 ounces short or medium grain white rice), 2¼ cups water, 1½ teaspoons salt

Batter: 6 ounces blended flours, 2¼ cups water, 1½ teaspoons salt
Warm with a target of 90°F (32°C) for 9 hours.

1st Feeding: 3 ounces blended flours
Warm with a target of 90°F (32°C) for 3 hours.

2nd Feeding: 3 ounces blended flours
Warm with a target of 90°F (32°C) for 3 hours.

Thicken or thin to taste, then cook at once in an oiled nonstick skillet or refrigerate for later.

Using blended flours also helps make the recipe more flexible. If you decide to experiment, you can easily swap other kinds of pulse and rice flour, homeground or commercial, for the ones I call for. You can also try different proportions, as dosa recipes can vary in ratio of rice to pulse from 4:1 to 1:1.

As I've warned more than once, though, avoid "sprouted" or "toasted" flours. Nowadays, such flours are popular especially for lentils and other pulses, because sprouting and toasting destroy lectins. But fermenting and cooking also do that, so you're covered.

Having trouble finding short or medium grain rice? Look in the bulk bins of your supermarket or natural foods store. Also, short grain rice is often sold as "sushi rice," while medium grain may be sold as "Calrose."

The most popular filling for dosa is potato curry, and the combination is common enough that it has its own name: *masala dosa*. It's traditionally meant for breakfast, but I personally can eat it for any meal, and it makes a perfect and very filling dinner by itself. I offer my own version here as Mark's Masala Dosa.

Preparation and cooking time for the curry alone is about one hour. This part of the recipe is based loosely on how I used to see it made by one of my hosts in India—but even so, I suspect it will make some Indian readers gasp in horror. The truth is, no self-respecting Indian cook would use anything called "curry powder," the spice combination I call for. Instead, they have a cupboard of individual spices they pick and combine themselves for each dish.

But my recipe does have one authentic and decidedly fun feature: You get to pop mustard seed like popcorn. With a glass pot top, you can watch the popping, while with a metal top, you can hear the seeds hitting it! Things can get a bit smoky, though, while you're waiting for the seeds to finish popping. So, ventilate as best you can, and if you have a sensitive smoke alarm, maybe disable it temporarily.

Despite being a long-time dosa fan, I'm far from an expert, so I urge you to look online for a multitude of other tips and recipes. And while you're there, maybe check out another Asian rice pancake that's traditionally fermented but which I haven't yet been brave enough to make: Vietnam's *banh xeo* (pronounced "bon say-o"). Then there's the sometimes fermented Indonesian rice pancake *dadar gulung*, with its spring-green coloring and coconut filling.

I'll have to find places to taste these before trying to make them, but my mouth is already watering!

Mark's Masala Dosa

About 3 cups batter for Smart Dosa
1 teaspoon mustard seeds
1 halved and sliced medium yellow onion
2 peeled and diced medium russet potatoes
1 cup water
2 teaspoons curry powder
1 teaspoon salt

1. Liberally oil the bottom of a large nonstick pot and add the mustard seeds.

2. Cover the pot securely. After ensuring good kitchen ventilation, place the pot on medium-high heat and wait for the seeds to pop. Do not leave the pot unattended!

3. As soon as the popping is done, lower the heat to medium. Carefully add the onion slices and then sauté till the half rings separate and become translucent.

4. Raise the heat back to medium-high and stir in the potatoes. Pour in the water, which should come to about half the height of the potatoes in the pot. Then stir in the curry powder and salt and again cover the pot.

5. When the water comes to a steady boil, lower the heat again to medium. Let the curry simmer for about a half hour, stirring occasionally and adding water if needed to prevent sticking. Continue till the potato pieces break down to roughly the consistency of mashed potatoes. Then remove the pot from the heat.

6. With the curry still warm (or rewarmed), make dosa of at least 6 inches (15 centimeters) in diameter. Place each dosa upside down on a plate and spoon some curry onto it in a column running from top edge to bottom. Roll the dosa around the curry and serve with the seam side down.

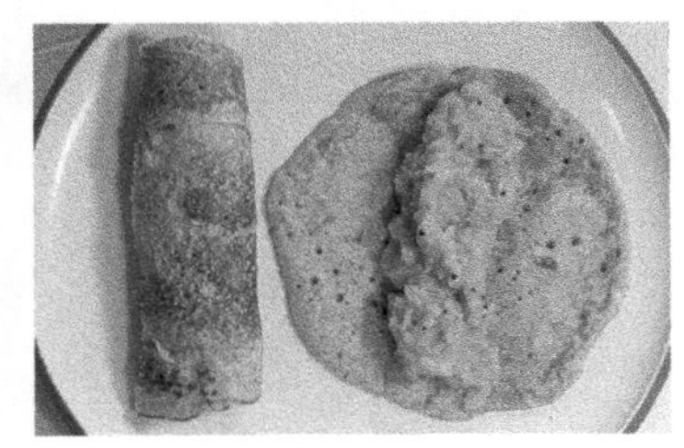

Beyond Sourdough

As popular as sourdough is nowadays, it's far from the only fermented food gaining interest. Also in the spotlight are a wide range of *probiotic* foods, with beneficial living microbes that contribute to the rich ecosystems in our digestive tracts.

These foods include relatively new favorites like yogurt—when it's not pasteurized—and older favorites like pickles and sauerkraut—when they're naturally fermented instead of made with vinegar. It's easy to buy such foods today. But it's also easy to make your own! And if you go that route—or are already traveling it—you might wonder if you can apply any lessons from smart sourdough.

I wondered that, myself. And my experiments have shown you can.

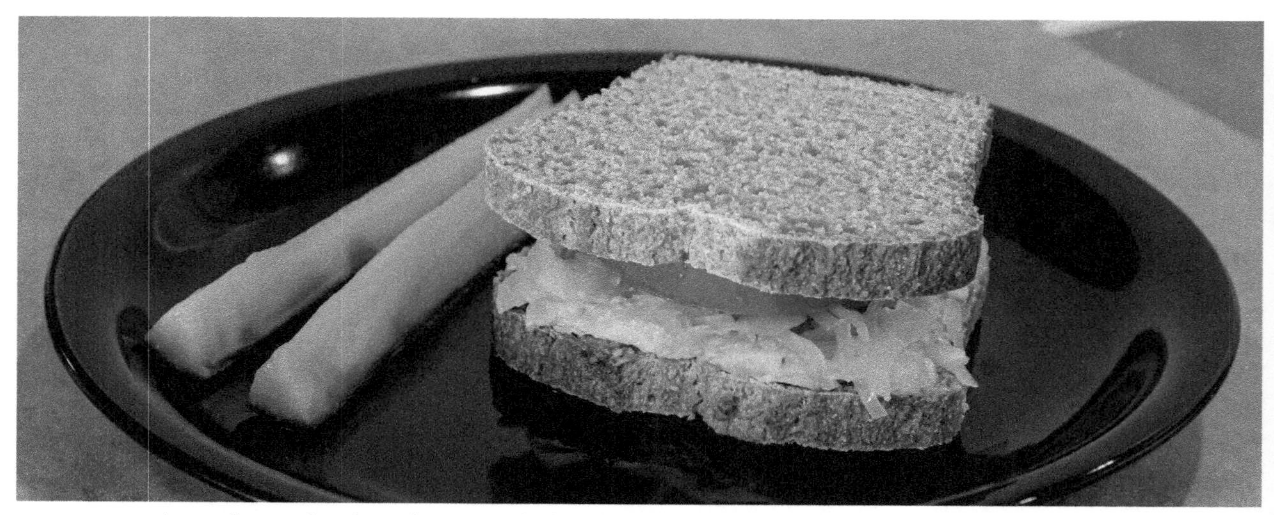

Avocado sandwich with 100% whole wheat smart sourdough and naturally fermented sauerkraut, with naturally fermented dill pickles on the side

For instance, most yogurt recipes tell you to first scald the milk at 180°F or so (around 85°C) to sterilize it and to help the yogurt thicken. And nearly all the rest tell you to heat the milk to an optimum temperature—generally 113°F (45°C)—*before* adding your yogurt starter.

Is any of that really needed? When I make a sponge of flour, water, and salt for my sourdough, nothing is preheated. Why should it be different for a mixture of yogurt and fresh pasteurized milk?

And in fact, I found I could take a quart of whole milk straight from the refrigerator, mix in a couple of spoonfuls of yogurt, put the whole thing in a wide mouth Mason jar in my proofer at a setting of 100°F (38°C), and have nicely thickened yogurt overnight. (The Mason jar acts like a little greenhouse, raising the temperature by about another ten degrees Fahrenheit.)

Of course, yogurt and smart sourdough are both fermented at high temperature, so you'd expect some techniques to work for both. But what about pickles? I'd made those occasionally for decades, naturally fermenting them at room temperature, which takes about three days.

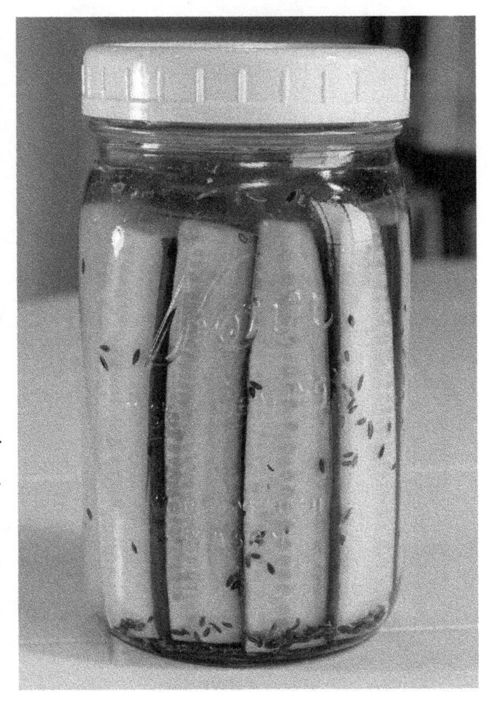

What would happen if my jar of cucumber spears, salt, dill seeds, and water was instead warmed in the proofer? Here's what: At a target temperature of 100°F (38°C)—with a setting of 95°F on my second-generation Brød & Taylor—I had delicious pickles in 24 hours! And I later had similar good results from a target of 110°F (43°C) with a proofer setting of 100°F.

Now we come to what some call the king of ferments—sauerkraut. I've been addicted to the naturally fermented variety ever since my very first taste of Bubbies Sauerkraut—the avowed entry drug for many of us sauerkraut lovers. And that's after nearly a lifetime of *hating* the standard commercial stuff made with vinegar.

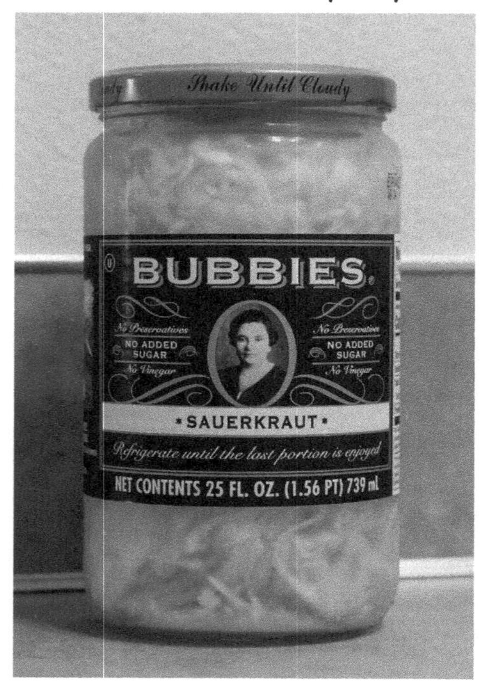

My dedication to sauerkraut was cemented when I noticed something unexpected about my teeth: Eating sauerkraut daily, I stopped getting cavities—*completely*—though I'd been getting them often before that. It's been several years now, and in that time, *I have not had a single cavity*. What's more, since starting to mix a tiny amount of sauerkraut juice with my evening orange juice, I've had noticeably less buildup of dental plaque—always a big problem for me before.

Think the connection with sauerkraut is far fetched? Look online for scientific studies of probiotics and tooth decay. Though you may not find a direct mention of sauerkraut, you will definitely see the names of lactic acid bacteria that ferment it.

Despite my love of sauerkraut, it took me a while to make any of my own, intimidated as I was by the messy preparation and long fermentation. Pickles were so much easier! But during a time when I had trouble getting my beloved Bubbies, I finally broke down and gave it a try.

The process wasn't as much trouble as I'd imagined, even with cutting the cabbage by hand, but my first results were disappointing. After being left on my kitchen counter for a week—

the advised minimum—the cabbage had fermented, but the taste was not good. The room temperature of my apartment was just too high above sauerkraut's recommended range.

Then I thought: There's no good way for me to lower the fermenting temperature. What if I push it higher?

So, I gave the sauerkraut the same treatment as my pickles, warming the jar in my proofer to a target temperature of 100°F (38°C). Sure enough, I had sauerkraut in 24 hours—and it tasted great! The flavor was milder than the norm, with more lactic acid and less acetic, but the pH was down to an impressive 3.5—more than low enough for all the health and practical benefits of sauerkraut. And later, a target temperature of 110°F (43°C) even gave me a more sour taste.

Want to learn more about making your own probiotics? Look for the many fine books and websites on home fermenting now available. So far, for myself, I've enjoyed books by Sandor Ellix Katz, Kirsten and Christopher Shockey, Kathryn Lukas and Shane Peterson, Holly Howe, Holly Davis, and Shannon Stonger. (For a truly encyclopedic overview, see Sandor Ellix Katz's *The Art of Fermentation.*)

Frequently Asked Questions

Isn't calling your method "smart sourdough" a bit presumptuous? It's like saying all other methods are not *smart.*

Actually, I'm playing off the title of a popular book series by my wife, Anne L. Watson—Smart Soapmaking—and the moniker has worked well for us there. It refers to the fact that a lot of what goes on in soapmaking is based on obsolete and incorrect ideas—and I feel that goes for sourdough too.

It's not that traditional methods don't work. It's just that they're a lot more complex and time consuming than they need to be—and that sets people up for failure. My method is much simpler, and once you've worked out a proper setup, it succeeds every time.

If you're adapting the principles of Type II sourdough, why not just call it that?

Besides it being a dorky name for a home method, Type II is, strictly speaking, an industrial process tailored to industrial supplies and equipment. For one thing, the flour is *not* fermented from scratch. Instead, Type II uses commercial starter that's not available to home bakers.

The only microbes in this commercial starter are isolated species of thermophilic ("heat-loving") bacteria—just as in starters for commercial yogurt. This allows heating to 45°C (113°F)—perfect for those bacteria, but too high for many species we want to nurture at home.

How can you be so sure that early yeast activity in a sponge or starter is from baker's yeast instead of wild yeast?

Because I got tricked by this myself when I began experiments for this book. That was during a period when my wife was baking yeast bread regularly. At first, my overnight sponges were bubbly and yeasty, and my bread rose wonderfully without my adding any yeast to the loaf.

But when my wife stopped baking her bread, the amount of yeast hanging around our home gradually declined. My sponges bubbled less and less, till they stopped doing that entirely. That's when I realized I'd been kidding myself—just as I believe many bakers do.

Did you really test all your recipes and variations on all your featured warming devices?

No, I can't claim that. I used all the featured warming devices to develop and test my basic recipe. Once I was satisfied with those results, I used my second-generation Brød & Taylor proofer for all other testing.

Your method doesn't sound that different from how I make yogurt. Can I just use a yogurt maker for my sourdough?

You'd think so, but I haven't found any yogurt maker I could easily adapt to my method. One problem is the small capacity of yogurt makers. The other is that most are designed to heat milk to 45°C (113°F). Add to that the heat generated by the sourdough bacteria themselves, and you're into the danger zone for many species.

The Yogurt Normal setting of the Instant Pot targets 40°C (104°F), which is low enough, and the device has enough room at least for a sponge. But that's with direct heating from a strong element with a wide swing of temperatures. That will create hot spots that will ruin your sourdough.

I often use Mason jars for fermenting vegetables and making yogurt. Can I use one in place of a bowl for my sourdough sponge?

I tried that for a while, using different jar coverings and even a vacuum pump, but I kept getting failures from runaway microbe activity. I'm not sure why. Maybe the tall shape lent itself to uneven heating. Anyway, I recommend sticking with a bowl.

Why would I need a proofer from Brød & Taylor when I can build my own?

Though it might be possible to build a homemade proofer for smart sourdough, most available designs won't work. Many rely on direct heating, which can create hot spots in your sponge and ruin it. Others simply won't give high enough temperatures.

Remember, you want to be able to gradually heat water to 100°F (38°C), then keep it there without wide swings. The Brød & Taylor achieves this with an absolute minimum of hassle. (And no, I have no financial interest in the company—I'm just a huge, grateful fan.)

You mention small loaf pans meant for ¾-pound loaves, but where can I find one? I've looked everywhere!

They're certainly rare nowadays, but I've seen them sold by online restaurant suppliers. Of course, you can always make a round loaf of the same size.

You don't recommend kneading with a food processor. But for those of us who want or need to do that anyway, do you have any tips?

Since I have no experience with it, I yield the floor to my wife, Anne L. Watson:

"You *can* knead dough with a food processor—if you have the right food processor. Check your manual, but also be aware that your manufacturer may give rather optimistic instructions. It takes a fairly powerful machine to knead dough, and if what you have is a light one that's better suited to slicing vegetables, you can burn out the motor. So, go cautiously. The first time, process your dough in two or more batches, listening for the sound of the machine straining.

"Use the steel blade—if your food processor came with a plastic one for kneading bread, ignore it. Those things may be good for something, but whatever it is, it's not bread.

"Use the machine very briefly, probably less than a minute. You want your dough mixed thoroughly, but it's easy to overdo it. As soon as it forms a smooth ball, that's enough.

"Take it carefully out of the machine. Knead it lightly by hand to see how it feels. If it's elastic and slightly sticky, it's ready.

"Oh, and don't even try kneading 100% rye dough. I ruined one food processor that way!"

How do I know my tap water is hot enough to kill all microbes left in my mixing bowl or on my kitchen spoon?

It's probably not—and it doesn't need to be. Killing all microbes is *sterilizing*. For sourdough, all you generally need to do with your equipment is *sanitize* it—kill enough of the microbes so they can't compete with the ones you want.

Your tap water should do this even at a water heater's lowest recommended setting—120°F (about 50°C)—if the water is allowed a little time to work. (Most water heaters are set higher than that, which will let the water kill more microbes more quickly but can also cause scalding burns and infant deaths.)

Of course, this assumes that your water is up to the temperature that's been set. It might be cooler, for instance, if you've just taken a shower, or if the water has traveled through cold pipes. You can always check with a thermometer.

I was late getting my sponge started, but I still need to have bread by a certain time. Is there any way to catch up?

Most warming devices take a couple of hours to bring the sponge up to your target temperature. If yours is like that, you could catch up by raising the temperature setting a little at the beginning—as long as you don't forget to lower it again before the sponge overheats! You could also warm your sponge a bit in a microwave—very carefully, and of course, not in a metal bowl. But don't try any of this without a decent thermometer.

Another option is just to accept having a shorter cycle time. That could be for the first cycle only, or you could split the difference between two or more cycles. By the end, your bread might be slightly less sour, but it would still be tasty, and you might not even notice the difference.

You could also redivide your remaining flour to give you one less feeding cycle. That might mean, for example, switching from a four-cycle sourdough to a three-cycle. Again, you'd lose some sourness, but you'd still get fine bread.

You suggest "rebaking" to restore stale loaves. How is that done?

Though I've seen a number of methods suggested online, I've only begun experimenting with it myself—mostly to revive loaves I've made for testing and then had to freeze because I had too much bread on hand! So far, I've had best results with this method: Stand the loaf on its cut end on an unoiled baking sheet, then bake at the same temperature for maybe ten to fifteen minutes less than originally. I'm aiming at an internal temperature of about 135°F (57°C), but I don't really have that nailed down yet as the optimum.

To keep the crust from getting so hard, you might try spritzing water on it with a mister before baking, or bagging the loaf before it cools completely.

Why don't you provide measurements in grams and liters along with ounces and cups?

I tried that at first, but I found myself approximating the conversions to round the measurements and make them easily divisible. Sticking with the same units I used to develop the recipes gave me greater accuracy and more consistency. I also found that conversions added a great deal of clutter to my recipe sketches, making them much less reader friendly.

At the same time, all modern digital scales can display in ounces as well as grams, and most fluid measuring cups and jugs are now graduated in cups as well as liters. So, providing conversions in a cookbook, I decided, was no longer essential. In fact, with the continuing rise of international cooking, I suspect it will go the way of the dodo.

How can you pretend that measuring in ounces instead of grams is precise enough for modern baking?

Measuring in *full* ounces is probably not. But please note I tell you that your digital scale needs to measure to a *tenth* of an ounce. When I then say, for example, to use 12 ounces of flour, that number should be understood as 12.0—and that's more than accurate enough for sourdough.

Measuring in grams, on the other hand, might give the impression of being more scientific, but that would really just be an illusion. You can't pin down sourdough that exactly.

How can you get sandwich bread with such high hydration?

The hydration—normally figured as the percentage of the liquid's weight against the flour's weight in the recipe—is not as high for my bread as it looks. That's because you have a good deal of evaporation at these high temperatures—up to half a cup by the time you shape the loaf—not to mention my adding a wild card ingredient, "extra flour for kneading." So, despite the amounts in my recipe, the hydration should be in a range typical of sandwich bread—around 67%, give or take.

Why don't you say up front that your book is mostly about whole wheat sourdough?

On the one hand, many people today take an automatic scunner to anything labeled "whole wheat," even when they would otherwise like it just fine. So, it's common for natural foods restaurants and bakeries to say nothing about that and just let their customers enjoy. I figured I should do the same.

On the other hand, many hard-core natural foodies don't consider a bread whole wheat unless it's 100%. The paltry 50% in my basic recipe just wouldn't cut it. By relinquishing the claim, I avoid riling the faithful. (Curiously, though, no one expects rye bread to be 100% rye.)

Will your baking method give me the crisp crust so prized by artisan bakers?

I can't say it will—or that I'd want it to. Speaking as an oldster with aging teeth, I can do without the heavy chewing needed to get through a typical artisan crust, however nice a photo it makes. If you have kids, they can probably do without it, too.

And don't get me started on bits of things spread on the crust, like seeds and cornmeal, that are hard enough to cause dental damage. Or on flour dustings that require ten minutes of cleanup after cutting a slice from the loaf.

Why do you focus on sandwich bread instead of artisan bread like all the other sourdough authors?

Because I believe most bread nowadays is eaten in sandwiches—as it is in my own diet. And the uneven slices and hard crusts of artisan loaves are just less practical for that. For me, sourdough isn't a delicacy, it's a staple—and I want it to be the same for more people.

Some artisan bakers too are waking up to the fact that their refined aesthetics are limiting acceptance of their bread. Search online for "Approachable Loaf."

You say not to insert your thermometer in the sponge till the end of a feeding cycle to avoid disturbing the surface. Is there any safe way to check temperature at other times?

An infrared thermometer won't work, because it measures temperature only at the surface, and underneath that, the sponge will be warmer. But you might try an aquarium thermometer, with the sensor left under the sponge at the center of the bowl. Sadly, I did not think of this until my recipe had been perfected and I was far along with this book.

Why do temperatures in the Brød & Taylor proofer jump a few degrees when I change the setting from 95°F to 96°F (or 35°C to 36°C)?

This happens *only* with their second-generation proofer—the current model, with a separate Proofer Mode. When designing this model, the company figured its customers *always* use steam from the water tray with settings up to 95°F (35°C). Since the steam raises the temperature of anything in the proofer about five degrees Fahrenheit (about three degrees Celsius), they compensated by reducing the heat from the proofer itself.

The compensation, though, stops right at 95°F (35°C)—because Brød & Taylor figured its customers *never* use the water tray *above* that setting. So, if you set the proofer just one degree higher, it reverts to normal levels of heating, making the temperature of anything in it jump by several degrees. This creates a gap that's smack in the middle of the proofer's range, with temperatures the proofer *cannot reach*.

Arbitrary? Frustrating? Confusing? Yes, it can be all of those. On the other hand, it *can* make temperature settings a little simpler—*if* you're using the proofer the way Brød & Taylor believes you are!

Is there any way to grind flour myself so the bran can be sifted out for a better rise?

If you're using a low-speed grain grinder and a softer wheat berry—like hard winter wheat instead of hard spring or hard white—your bran *might* flake off in pieces large enough for at least partial removal with a 40-mesh flour sifter. This *might* improve your rise. (It would also slightly reduce the flour weight.)

Your No-Rise Pancakes—why don't you just call them crepes?

I had meant to, but my wife assured me they were nothing of the sort. Crepes are made thinner with batters that include milk and eggs. Even using a crepe maker, my wife could not get the thinness she wanted with my recipe.

You mentioned that Indians make dosa with "urad dal" and "idli rice." What are those exactly? And if I want to try them, where can I find them?

Urad dal, though little known in the United States, has many names worldwide, including *black gram*. The kind used for dosa can be either split or whole, but in either case, it's normally "skinned," with the black hulls removed. This kind is pale colored and is often called "white" urad dal.

Idli rice is a parboiled short or medium grain white rice. (*Idli* may also be spelled *idly*.) Just don't buy *idli rava* (cream of rice) or an idli mix, which has other ingredients added. And don't confuse idli rice with the "converted rice" made in the United States, which is likewise parboiled but is long grain instead.

You should be able to find these at Indian markets and from online retailers. With the white urad dal, though, be careful about freshness. Skinning leaves it more liable to spoil, and since it comes from India for specialty use only, some suppliers may have it sitting around for quite some time. (Buying imported flour is even riskier.)

For myself, I found I got tastier dosa from my lentils and plain rice!

Are there any important microbes in sourdough besides the yeast and lactic acid bacteria you talk about?

As I was finishing up this book, the Global Sourdough Project reported on their study of five hundred starters from around the world. The big surprise was that almost a third of those starters featured acetic acid bacteria as well as the yeast and lactic acid bacteria already well known to contribute. With many of those starters, this made the bread notably more sour in taste and slower to rise.

But I doubt acetic acid bacteria are ever that important in smart sourdough, as their preferred temperature range is well below what we use. So, they shouldn't need to concern us.

Is it true that vegans can get B_{12} from sourdough?

Some species of lactic acid bacteria produce vitamin B_{12}, an essential nutrient that can be hard to get in a vegan diet. Since each sourdough culture has its own blend of species—and since bacteria of any one species can act differently under different conditions—you can't assume just any sourdough bread will supply this vitamin or that it comes in a usable form. But the high fermenting temperatures of smart sourdough do favor species known to produce it.

How did you get to this new method from the one in your first sourdough book, Simple Sourdough*?*

After publishing that book, I discovered that beginning a sourdough starter was much harder in some settings than in others. I'm still not sure why, but my theory is it has something to do with the relative humidity of homes heated by gas and electric heat. (Electric heat is much "drier" than the gas heat I had while learning to make sourdough and while writing that first book.)

Anyway, the method in *Smart Sourdough* grew out of my efforts to find a more reliable way to launch a starter. In the end, my method was so reliable, I realized I didn't need a starter at all.

If adding salt early helps in fermenting a sponge, wouldn't it help the same way in a traditional sourdough starter?

That's my belief. In fact, I suspect that keeping salt out of starters is one reason so many attempts end in failure.

Few home fermenters would think of omitting salt when making pickles or sauerkraut, because that's just inviting bad microbes to grow. It's the salt that tips the balance toward success.

It's probably much the same with a sourdough starter. If I ever update my earlier book *Simple Sourdough*, I would hope to include a no-fail starter method—with salt.

Does your sourdough bread make good French toast?

Yes, indeed! I've had good results with a batter like what my mother, Lillian, used to make. The following ingredients make enough for most or all of a large loaf. (You might need a whisk for the cinnamon.)

- 1 cup whole milk
- 1 egg
- ¼ teaspoon salt
- ¼ teaspoon cinnamon (optional)

I thought Anne was married to a guy named Aaron!

She is! But for this book, I decided to stick to the name on my first book on sourdough, rather than the name I mostly use today. Don't worry, Anne's not a bigamist!

Are these really "frequently asked questions," or did you just make them up?

I've asked myself that, many times.

Sourdough vs. Salt-Rising

Aren't the high temperatures for smart sourdough the same as for salt-rising bread? And is that why it's smelling so bad?

Funny you should mention that! While winding up this book, I became aware that some of my early failures—as well as some odd results with a new brand of wheat berries I'm grinding—might be due less to the "runaway microbe activity" I've discussed and more to straying into the territory of salt-rising bread.

For the sake of the uninitiated, salt-rising is a fermented bread originally popular in America's Appalachian Mountains. But the bacteria that ferment it aren't the usual suspects—they're from the species *Clostridium perfringens*, most likely along with other, similar species.

These "salt-rising bacteria" are salt-tolerant and heat-loving but otherwise very different from the lactic acid bacteria that give us sourdough. For one thing, they can form dormant spores that survive even the heat of cooking and are in fact activated by it. They like things alkaline instead of acid. They feed mainly on the grain's protein rather than its starch (which makes for fairly dense bread). And they are very fast-growing.

Salt-rising bacteria are also distinguished by their waste products. The gas that puts the *rising* in "salt-rising"—and that can be seen in a sponge as strong fizzing or doming—is hydrogen rather than carbon dioxide. And the acids they produce are less lactic and acetic and more butyric and propionic. It's these two acids that give salt-rising bread the stinky cheese smell that some people love but many hate. (This family of bacteria also gives us the toxins associated with botulism and gangrene—but for whatever reason, they don't do that in bread dough.)

Like sourdough bacteria, salt-rising bacteria are abundant in whole grain flour, as well as in nature in general. But in sourdough, they're normally held in check by those sourdough bacteria and the acids they produce. To make salt-rising bread, then, you want to *kill off* the sourdough bacteria.

This is typically done by boiling the water or scalding the milk, then mixing it still hot in the sponge. Actually, the liquid's high heat kills off *all* active microbes in the flour—including salt-rising bacteria—but at the same time, it activates the dormant salt-rising *spores*, which then germinate and *become* active. After that, you just maintain the high fermenting temperatures these bacteria love, and with nothing to stand in their way, they quickly take over.

The problem is, with the high temperatures of smart sourdough, you may sometimes nurture the salt-rising bacteria without meaning to. This can happen if you let the sourdough bacteria run low on food before they produce enough acid to discourage their salt-rising rivals. Or it can happen if you use strong heating methods like direct heating that create hot spots in your sponge. Or it can happen if your flour was milled at a temperature high enough to kill the active bacteria and activate the salt-rising spores.

If you carefully follow this book's instructions, you should avoid such situations. But in case you still encounter that infamous salt-rising aroma, here are some ways you might avoid it the next time:

- Make your sourdough with whole grain flour milled at a lower temperature, to make sure enough sourdough bacteria have survived. If you're buying the flour, that might mean getting a higher-quality brand. (You can't go wrong with the King Arthur flours I used for most testing.) If you're grinding your own, you can refrigerate the grain before grinding, grind smaller amounts, or grind at a coarser setting. Harder or larger berries may take more to keep cool while grinding.

• If your whole grain flour seems weak in sourdough bacteria, mix in a little flour that's stronger. Rye flour, for instance, is often less processed than wheat and richer in those bacteria.

• If your water is very alkaline, replace it with water that's less so. For instance, most commercial spring water is near neutral. (You can look online for the pH of specific brands.)

• Make sure your sponge temperatures haven't crept up with seasonal or other changes. For example, having no thermostat, the Brød & Taylor proofer is simply calibrated for use at typical room temperatures. On a hot summer day, in a kitchen without air conditioning, the proofer can bring your sponge to a higher temperature than it would in winter.

• Lower your target sponge temperature by a few degrees, at least for the first one or two feeding cycles. Though this will normally make your sourdough less sour, it can also remove some advantage of the salt-rising bacteria.

• If you're used to fermenting vegetables in a glass Mason jar, *don't* try this with your sponge. Radiant heat converts the jar to a mini-greenhouse—and as I discovered for myself, this generally leads to an explosion of salt-rising bacteria. (Fermenting grains, with their mix of starch and protein, is a little different from fermenting vegetables!)

• If you're experimenting with exotic ferments in your kitchen, keep their microbes away from your sourdough. The spore-forming *Bacillus subtilis*, for instance, might be great for fermenting soybeans, but it may act as salt-rising bacteria in your sponge. Preventing contamination might be as simple as covering a bowl of flour you set on your counter, or at the other extreme, you might have to wipe down or spray your equipment with 70% isopropyl alcohol. Best yet, if you want to make sourdough without starter, don't cultivate rival microbes in your kitchen!

• Add to your sponge a little brine from naturally fermented pickles or sauerkraut as a starter just for the bacteria. Other fermented foods might work as starters too, but make sure you know how they're made! For example, I once tried adding store-branded water kefir, mainly to see if its yeast would raise my bread. In the end, I had to conclude the kefir microbes were dead on arrival, and the only live culture in that bottle was a token post-ferment shot of *Bacillus subtilis*. Exactly what I did not want!

Of course, you might *like* to try salt-rising bread. You can learn much more about it from the book *Salt Rising Bread*, by Genevieve Bardwell and Susan Ray Brown.

Index

For recipes, please see the table of contents. Recipe ingredients are indexed only when appearing in background discussions or recipe tips.

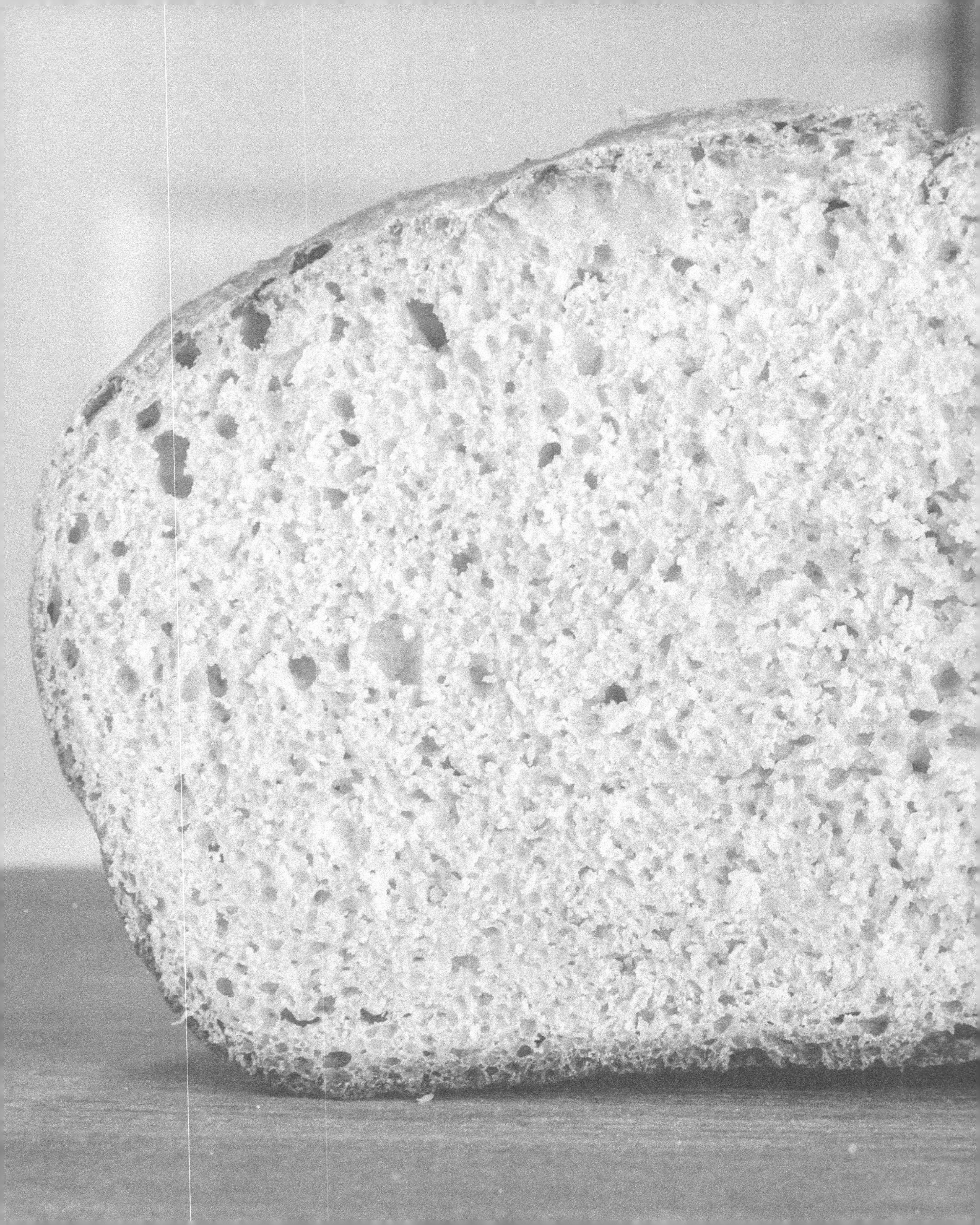

About the Author

Mark Shepard is the author of several books on simple living, nonviolent social change, and the flute, as well as children's books under the name Aaron Shepard. He first learned to love sourdough in 1979 while visiting the Community of the Ark, a utopian society founded in France by an Italian disciple of Mahatma Gandhi.

On Mark's return home, a friend taught him how to make sourdough of his own. After years of baking and devouring several loaves a week, he wrote and published the bestselling booklet *Simple Sourdough.*

Mark now lives in Bellingham, Washington, with his wife and fellow author, Anne L. Watson. Visit him at

www.markshep.com/sourdough

ALSO FROM SHEPARD PUBLICATIONS

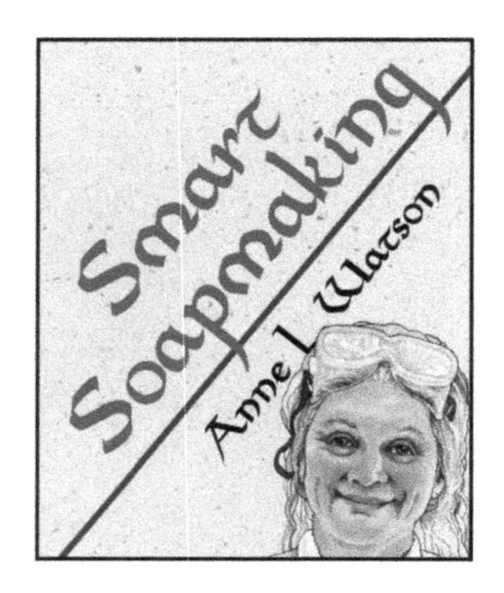

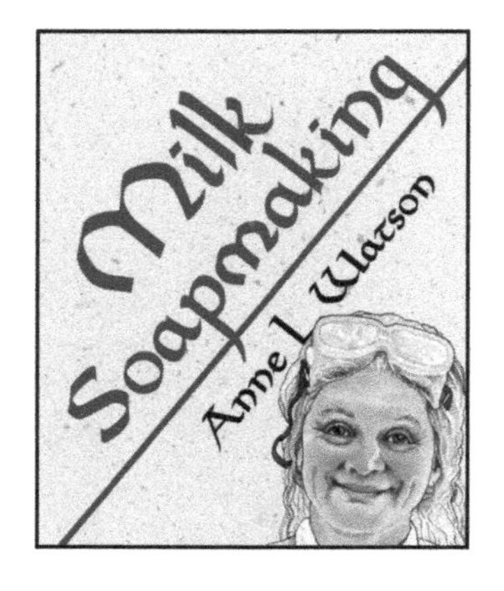

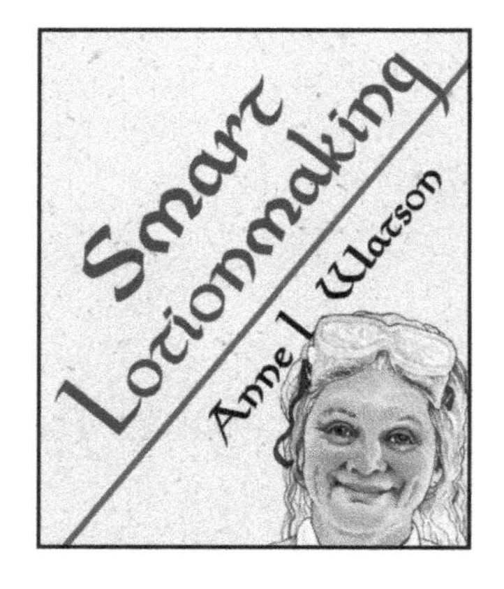

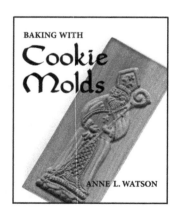

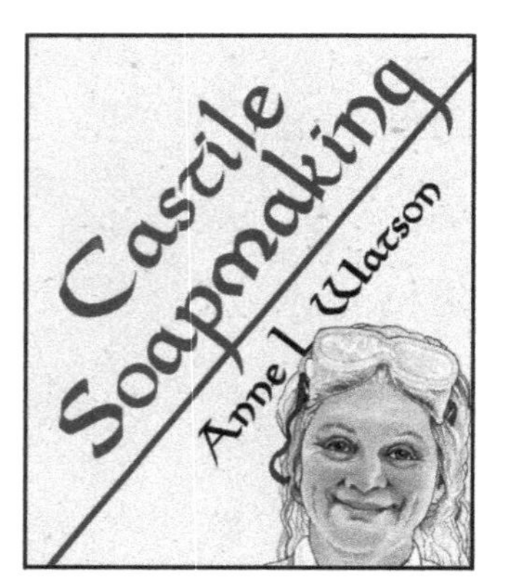

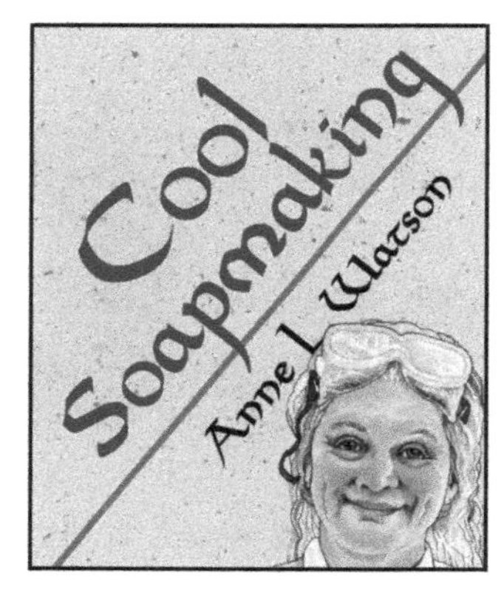

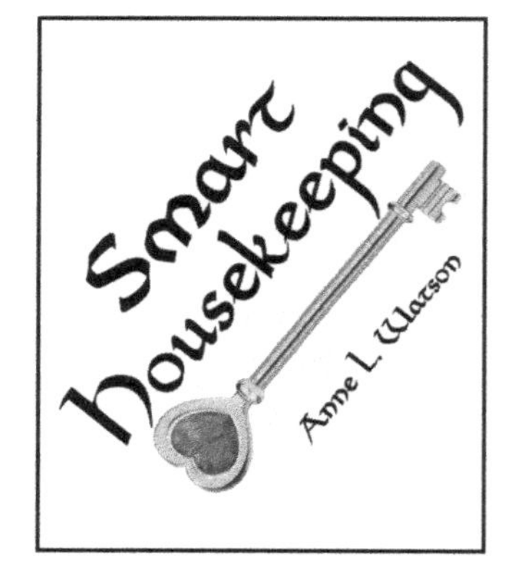

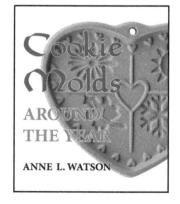

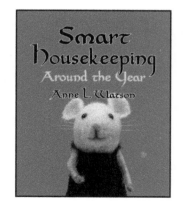

and more . . .

NOTES

CPSIA information can be obtained
at www.ICGtesting.com
Printed in the USA
BVHW021052041221
622872BV00022B/363